EVOLUTION OF AN
ACADEMIC DEPARTMENT

Evolution of an Academic Department

Obstetrics and Gynecology at the
University of South Florida

Barry S. Verkauf, MD, MBA

Library of Congress Control Number:		2013923317
ISBN:	Hardcover	978-1-4931-5628-3
	Softcover	978-1-4931-5627-6
	eBook	978-1-4931-5629-0

This book was printed in the United States of America.

Rev. date: 03/03/2014

To order additional copies of this book, contact:
Xlibris LLC
1-888-795-4274
www.Xlibris.com
Orders@Xlibris.com
542342

CONTENTS

PREFACE

Books are the material evidence of what we know. They represent knowledge, and through them, we discover what we know and who we are. Historical books present a chronological record of events. In this volume, I have told the story of an academic department in a medical school. Like most stories, some of the information is documented, but much information or knowledge is passed orally from one individual to another.

Undoubtedly, some information may be inadvertently omitted, and some information contained herein is subject to interpretation. It has not been my purpose to pass judgment on these events but, rather, to simply describe them in light of the times in which they occurred as I understood them. Many individuals have contributed to the complexion, highs, lows, foibles, and feats of the Department of Obstetrics and Gynecology at the University of South Florida Morsani College of Medicine. But my principal purpose here has been to describe the evolution of the organization as a whole and those who set the direction of its future.

An organization is a social arrangement among individuals, which pursues collective goals, controls its own performance, and has a boundary separating it from its environment. Like the individuals who comprise it, the organization reactively or proactively responds to the needs and the exigencies of the external environment that surrounds it. That environment in the twentieth century—particularly its last half and on into the present—has been one of increasingly rapid change. Alvin Toffler, in his 1970 book *Future Shock*,[1] expressed doubt regarding man's psychological capacity to adapt successfully to the rapidity of coming change and indicated that it would challenge organizations as well.

---

[1]   Alvin Toffler, *Future Shock* (Bantam Books, 1970).

It has often been said that "change is a constant." Like in the eons that have passed, adaptability to change is necessary for survival. This book is the story of that adaptation as it relates to a particular type of organization—the Department of Obstetrics and Gynecology in a medical school.

Departments in medical schools are hierarchical in nature. They are also matrix organizations in which each member serves two different hierarchies. One hierarchy is functional. It ensures that each expert or member of the various divisions or sections of the organization is well trained and monitored by a division head, who is often a "super expert" in the same field and who leads projects for which a particular division or unit has responsibility. The other is executive in nature—envisioning and getting products and projects completed by the experts. Ultimately, this executive function is usually the responsibility of the chairman of the department. It requires sensing the needs of the individuals within it and of the external environment and, often, ensuring adaptation to those needs to enable the success of the organization as a whole.

Organizations in medicine—and, therefore, physician training in medicine—have, of necessity, evolved constantly over the past forty years during the lifetime of the Department of Obstetrics and Gynecology at the University of South Florida Morsani College of Medicine. The need for adaptation has required capable leaders to recognize and implement needed change in order for their departments to survive and be successful. This book focuses upon those leaders, the timeliness of their presence, their unique skills, and their accomplishments.

January 25, 2011

Acknowledgments

Like most authors, I am indebted to a number of friends and colleagues, without whom this book would not have been possible. My thanks to those members of the Department of Obstetrics and Gynecology who contributed chapters and many other members of the department, both present and past, who shared their knowledge and remembrances with me. Because much of the background of this book is from collective memory, there may be certain inaccuracies, for which I take responsibility, as well as interpretations of the recorded background described on which the departmental change took place. While the book is best read in its entirety, each chapter is written to stand alone.

La Tasha Morgan and Cindy Smith are responsible for much of the organizational work in bringing this book to completion, and for that, they have my sincere appreciation. My thanks go as well to Linda Potocki for typing and retyping the manuscript. I am indebted to Athar Naif for skillfully gathering and recording information regarding the percentage of USF students who have entered obstetrics and gynecology as a specialty, and to Wanda Rodriguez and Lauren Shaw for collecting information regarding residents under each of the three departmental chairmen.

I am fortunate to have had the counsel of Bruce Shephard, MD; J. K. Williams, MD; Cathy Lynch, MD; and Elaine Shimberg—all accomplished medical authors—both for direction and for reviewing the manuscript. And, of course, I want to express my thanks to the University of South Florida for the privilege and opportunity to write about it.

List of Contributors

Larry Glazerman, MD, MBA
Associate Professor and Director
Division Director of Minimally Invasive Surgery

Mitchel Hoffman, MD
Teasley-Tampa General Professor and Division Director
Division of Gynecologic Oncology

Lennox Hoyte, MD, MSEE
Associate Professor and Director
Division of Urogynecology

Stephen Klasko, MD, MBA
Professor, VP for USF Health, and Dean of Morsani College of Medicine
Division of General Obstetrics and Gynecology

Catherine Lynch, MD
Interim Chair, Professor, and Director
Division of General Obstetrics and Gynecology

Michael T. Parsons, MD, MBA
Professor
Division of Maternal-Fetal Medicine

Shayne Plosker, MD
Associate Professor and Director
Division of Reproductive Endocrinology and Infertility

John Tsibris, PhD
Professor and Director
Division of Research

Barry Verkauf, MD, MBA
Professor
Division of Reproductive Endocrinology and Infertility

J. K. Williams, MD
Professor and Director
Division of Gynecologic Specialties
Evolution of an Academic Department

The Department of Obstetrics and
Gynecology at the University of South Florida

Celebrating the First Forty Years

Barry S. Verkauf, MD, MBA

Introduction to Chapter 1

The Age of Innocence

Once upon a time, not so long ago, in a place not so far away, the practice of medicine was relatively simple and, for physicians, very sweet. While the 1950s and 1960s had seen the bitter battle over the passage and implementation of Medicare and Medicaid, that time had passed, and physicians were now paid by the government for providing care to the elderly and poor, which they often used to do freely and for no compensation. The supply of physicians did not yet meet the demand for their services, and a young doctor could "hang up his shingle" just about anywhere and count on earning a living.

Virtually everyone still knew a friend or family member injured in the Second World War, Korean War, or Vietnam War, and the value of physicians in wartime—as well as their ethical posture in peacetime—had set them on a pedestal. War always brings scientific advances, which are transformed into civilian life, bettering the health and living standards of the civilian population. Physicians were the most respected segment of society. Their authority was rarely questioned by patients or third-party payers and insurance companies, which by this time were participants in the economics of medical practice. Technological and scientific advance was rapid, making work for the physician challenging but exciting to embrace. Times were good for those entering the medical profession.

Moreover, the United States was still competing with the Soviet Union for primacy in the world. Federal funding for scientific research and training of new physicians was still relatively abundant. While the decade of 1974–1984 brought the first oil crisis the United States had ever seen, with cars waiting in line for gas and with subsequent inflation and slow economic growth (stagflation) and two recessions, Florida fared better than the rest of the country during this vexing time. Migration into Florida and growth within the state continued at a reasonable pace. It was under these circumstances that the Department of Obstetrics and Gynecology at the University of South Florida had its beginnings.

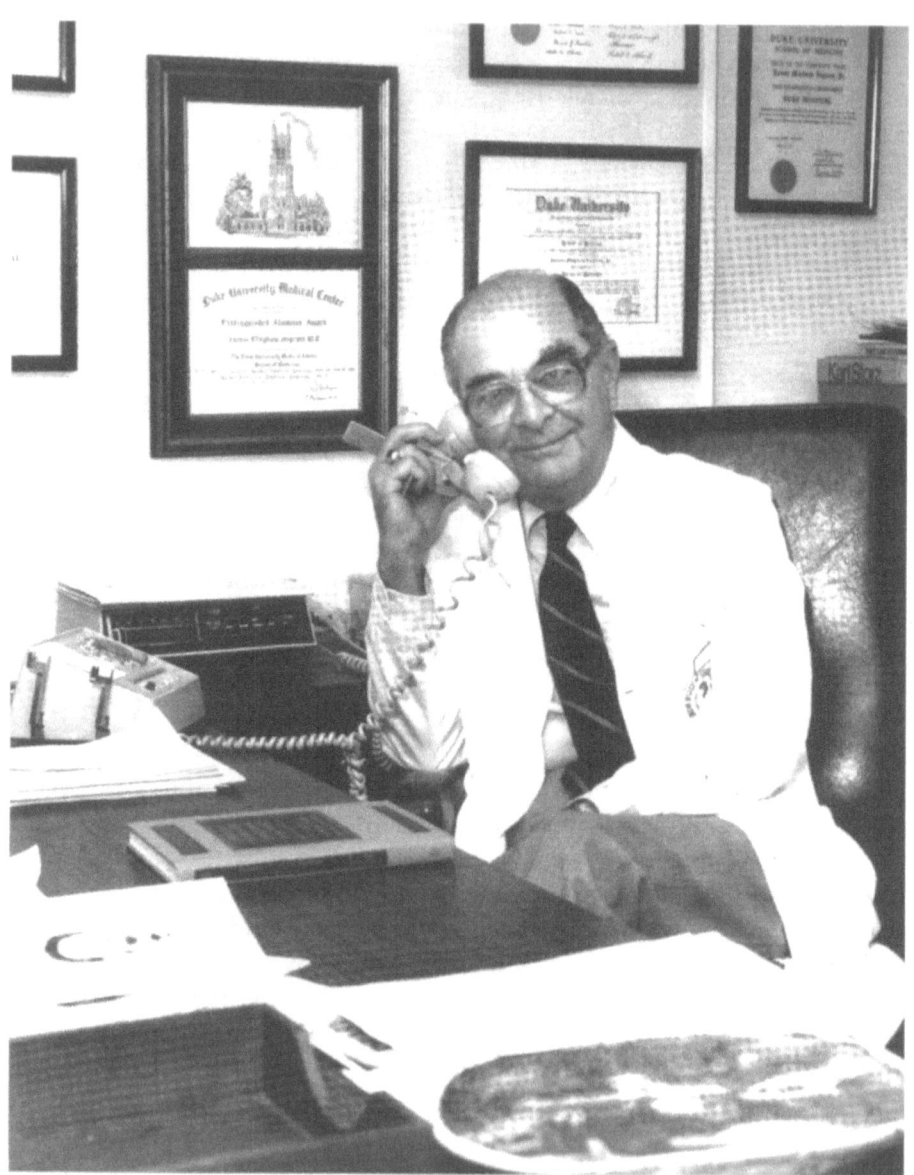

Dr. Ingram at his desk

CHAPTER 1

James Mayhew Ingram Jr., MD

by Barry S. Verkauf, MD, MBA

James Mayhew Ingram Jr. was born in Bessemer, Alabama, in 1921. He moved to Tampa during his early boyhood years when his father entered into the orange-grove business. The groves they owned were in the area now known as Carrollwood. Young Jim Jr. went to elementary and secondary schools through the public school system in Tampa, attended the University of Tampa for two years, and graduated from Duke University in 1940. After graduating from college, he attended Duke University School of Medicine, receiving his degree as a doctor of medicine in 1944 and graduating with the distinction of earning admission to Alpha Omega Alpha Honor Medical Society.

Dr. Ingram subsequently served a year of internship in medicine at the Johns Hopkins Hospital in Baltimore but returned to Duke to begin a residency in obstetrics and gynecology late in 1944. In 1946, he was drafted into the US Army, where he spent two years at Walter Reed Army Medical Center in Washington, DC, and then as chief of obstetrics and gynecology at an army hospital in Puerto Rico. Discharged as a captain in 1948, he returned to Duke to complete his residency in obstetrics and gynecology, which he did in 1951, serving as the chief resident-instructor at Duke University Hospital in Durham. During this interval, he spent six months at the Johns Hopkins Hospital, studying gynecologic pathology under the direction of Emil Novak, the Father of Gynecologic Pathology. It was here that Dr. Ingram began his academic interests and initiated his first publication (Ingram and Novak 1951, 61:774), which was a seminal paper on the relationship between endometrial carcinoma and feminizing ovarian tumors.

DR. EMIL NOVAK
26 EAST PRESTON STREET
BALTIMORE-2, MD

March 18, 1950

Dr. James Ingram
Department of Obstetrics and Gynecology
Duke Hospital
Durham, North Carolina

Dear Jim:

I am sure you must have been wondering as to what disposition had been made of our paper, but to be perfectly frank I had hesitated about sending it in to the American Journal for the simple reason that I had a paper in that publication only recently, and another one is due in the near future. I was afraid that my friend, George Kosmak, might think it rather piggish of me to want another one published so soon.

Since you were good enough to give me disposal of the paper I have had it placed on the program of the American Association of Obstetricians and Gynecologists, which meets in September, as presentation of the paper at that meeting will automatically insure its publication in the American Journal. I thought it best to do this in spite of the delay.

Incidentally the photomicrograph of one of our cases (I believe it is Case I, but I do not have the paper at hand as I dictate this letter) has never seemed to me to carry a great deal of conviction, and if, after I go over the slides again, it seems best to omit this case, I trust that this will be agreeable to you.

We miss you at the hospital and in the laboratory, but I am sure that you are getting a lot of fine work at Duke. Eddie is now on the home stretch, and getting a lot of good operative experience.

I am of course looking forward to his coming into practice with me in July.

Give my best regards to Drs. Carter, Ross and all my other good friends at Duke.

With the best of good wishes, I am

Very sincerely,

Emil Novak

EN:C

Letter to Dr. Ingram in 1950 from Dr. Emil Novak

Upon completing his residency in obstetrics and gynecology, despite the need for physicians in post–World War II America, there seemed to be few job opportunities in Tampa, where he desired to return. He entered private practice as the island physician in general medicine in Boca Grande, Florida, for a short period of time before joining Dr. Robert Withers—who also trained at Duke in the practice of obstetrics and gynecology in Tampa—in 1951. They were subsequently joined by Dr. Henry Wright—who completed his residency at Tampa General Hospital—in the practice of Ingram, Withers, and Wright, which became a popular and prestigious one in the Tampa community.

Dr. Wright subsequently retired to Boca Grande to take a position there as island physician, which Dr. Ingram had previously held, and Dr. Withers later entered solo practice in the northern part of the city and was instrumental in the evolution of Florida Hospital Tampa, which currently exists at the corner of Fletcher and Bruce B. Downs.

Dr. Ingram maintained a practice in South Tampa and was subsequently joined by Drs. Robert Qualey and Byrne Marston, both trained at Case Western Reserve University, and soon after by Dr. Robert McCammon, trained at the University of Indiana. The practice of Ingram, Qualey, Marston, and McCammon similarly earned a prominent and influential position in the Tampa Bay area. While practicing private medicine in Tampa, Dr. Ingram held an appointment as clinical assistant professor in obstetrics and gynecology at the University of Florida College of Medicine in Gainesville.

Dr. Ingram was intuitively and politically astute and always the consummate diplomat (in the best sense of these words). He was heavily involved in medical academics and politics as they existed at the time. He was an early member of many medical societies, including the Bayard Carter Society, the South Central Obstetrical and Gynecological Society, the Continental Gynecologic Society, the Central Gynecologic Society, and the South Atlantic Association of Obstetricians and Gynecologists, the latter of which, at the time, was one of the most influential OB-GYN organizations in the country. Prior to the formation of the American Congress of Obstetricians and Gynecologists, it was societies such as these where academic and political leaders met to set the course and influence the direction of the specialty of obstetrics and gynecology. Dr. Ingram was president of almost every organization to which he belonged but seemed most sentimentally attached to the South Atlantic Association of Obstetricians and Gynecologists.

Locally, he was intimately involved in the Hillsborough County Medical Association and the Florida Obstetric and Gynecologic Society and, as usual, ultimately became president of each. He was also a member of the Florida Medical Association and served as the chairman of the committee on maternal health for Florida from 1960 to 1965 and on the board of governors for the Florida Medical Association from 1966 to '67.

He served on the board of directors at St. Joseph's Hospital in 1973–75 and chief of obstetrics and gynecology at Tampa General Hospital for over eight years. He was elected to several prestigious medical societies, including the American Association of Obstetrics and Gynecology and the American Gynecological Club. He was asked to serve as an examiner for the American Board of Obstetrics and Gynecology from 1974 through 1978 and was a director of this prestigious educational organization from 1979 through 1992. He received an Honorary Service Award from the University of Tampa, Duke University, and the University of South Florida.

In the early 1960s, substantial government funding was available to enhance medical research and education in the United States following the post–World War II baby boom. At that time, there were only two medical schools in the state—the University of Florida in Gainesville (a rural community at the time) and the state-supported medical school associated with the private University of Miami in the metropolitan area of Southeast Florida. The Tampa Bay region received attention as a natural site for a third medical school, and this unique opportunity generated great interest among local politicians and, particularly, the medical community. The Hillsborough County Medical Association appointed a committee on the medical school on which, from the beginning, Dr. Ingram served along with many other notable physicians from the community, including Dr. Woody York, Dr. Richard Connar, Dr. Irving Essrig, and Dr. Eugene Ruffolo, among others. With the need for trained physicians increasing after the Second World War, internships and residencies were available not only in academic institutional hospitals, but in community-hospital programs as well. This was true in Tampa, and a director for medical education was hired by Tampa General Hospital to coordinate these residency programs in this community. Dr. Ingram served as the point man and chief educator of the residents in OB-GYN by virtue of his energy and academic inclination.

While a new medical school would be on the campus of the University of South Florida in newly constructed facilities for a school there, the teaching in the clinical departments was to be accomplished principally by community physicians, who would provide their time and clinical expertise in training medical students in the clinical years, as well as residents. Dr. Ingram was heavily involved in all these discussions, and when the founding faculty of the medical school was introduced in 1970, consisting of nine people, Dr. Ingram had been appointed as chairman of OB-GYN, the only clinical department represented.

The residency program at Tampa General Hospital, already in existence for over fifteen years, served as the nucleus for the beginning of the clinical programs at the University of South Florida. Dr. Ingram, having heavily been involved for many years in the teaching of residents and in the political evolution of the medical school and with a national reputation

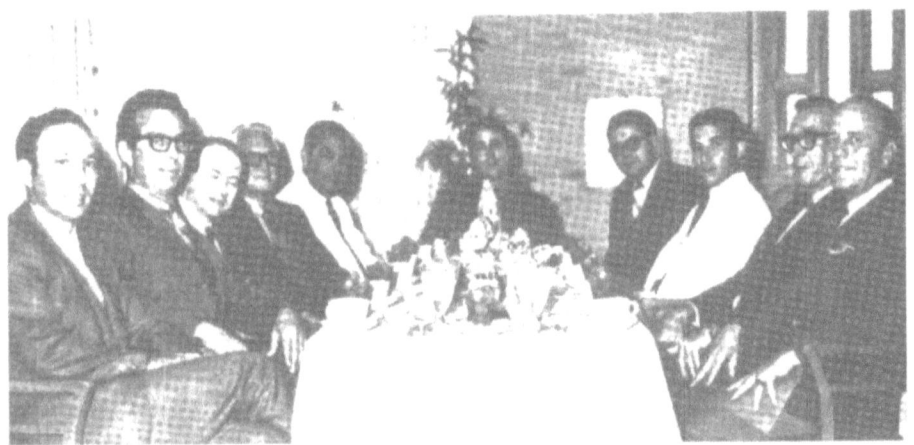

Original founding faculty of USF Medical School; Dr. Ingram fifth from left

and connections, seemed to be the right person in the right place and at the right time to become the first full-time chairman of obstetrics and gynecology. He eagerly took on these duties and expanded the department. He actually wrote letters to all members of the Tampa Bay obstetrical community, asking for their advice and help in fashioning the new program; almost all volunteered to be on his clinical faculty.

Dr. Ingram maintained good relationships throughout the medical community, including the university faculty, practicing physicians in the community, and residents and students. He was highly respected and liked by all, and there are many stories that abound regarding him. The residents like to recall that despite the fact that after 1964 he did not practice obstetrics, the one day of the year that he attended obstetrical rounds was on Christmas morning, always in corduroy pants with whales on them. He regularly held journal clubs at his own home in the evening, to which he invited clinical faculty from the community, as well as residents and students. Many Ingram aphorisms emanated from these journal clubs, such as the one recalled by one of his ex-residents: "A dog may be man's best friend, but panty hoses are woman's greatest enemy." During the Christmas season, he entertained all the residents at parties at his home on Robin Lane, which were always memorable.

Dr. Ingram's interests were not only political and academic. He was a highly skilled clinician as well. In his early years of private practice, he practiced both obstetrics and gynecology, while in his latter years and at the university, his practice was limited to gynecology. He had a particular interest in gynecologic surgery and was an innovative as well as a gifted surgeon. He had particular interest in the two clinical entities of stress urinary incontinence for which he devised the Ingram catheter (Ingram 1972, 113:1108; Sharpe and Ingram 1973, 110:340) used postoperatively for urinary drainage and in congenital absence of the vagina. The latter is an uncommon clinical entity for which two types of treatment altered cyclically in clinical popularity. The surgical approach, principally McIndoe's (1938, 45:490–494) split-thickness skin graft, which enhanced the efficacy of the Wharton (1938, 107:843–854) modification of the original Abbe (1898, 84:836) procedure, was popular during the 1960s and 1970s. A nonoperative approach using vaginal dilators, which put pressure against the perineum, devised by R. T. Frank (1938, 35:1053–1055), had fallen into disuse because of the inconvenience of applying pressure to the perineum to create a neovagina and the time required to do so.

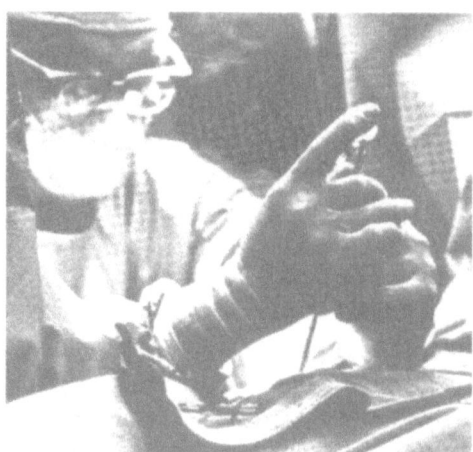

Dr. Ingram placing the Ingram catheter

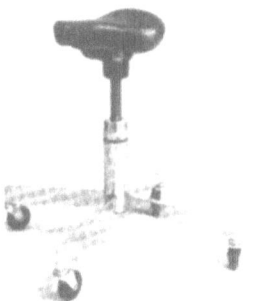

The Ingram bicycle seat

To meet this challenge, Dr. Ingram devised the Ingram bicycle seat (Ingram 1981, 140:8, 867–873). This was an ingenious innovation in which young women could sit on a bicycle seat attached to a rolling base on which pressure could be placed on the perineum with progressively larger Ingram dilators, allowing these young women to be mobile and facilitating the ease with which the nonoperative technique could be utilized. As time has progressed, the Ingram bicycle seat has grown in popularity, has been shown to be comparable to many operative methods in outcome, and generated some mirth at the time. When introduced at a distinguished assembly of California gynecologists, it was

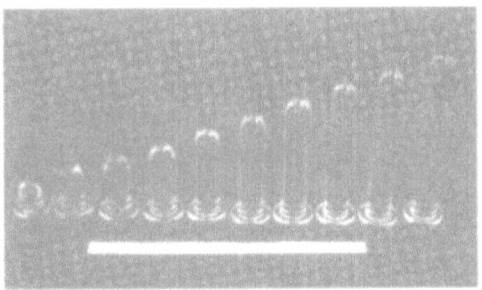

Ingram dilators used for creating a neovagina

with the following poem:

> There once was a girl name Regina
> Who was born without a vagina.
> She created such heat on her bicycle seat
> That she suffered an attack of angina.

Without a vagina, she'd retreat
From any new man she would meet.
But you made her more bold with her vaginal mold.
Now she's married her bicycle seat.

James Mayhew Ingram Jr. was an exceptional individual. Despite his many achievements as a practicing clinician, academic leader, and political force in medicine, he found time to be active in the Tampa social community as well. He belonged to several social clubs and civic organizations but was most active in Ye Mystic Krewe of Gasparilla of which he served as Lord Chamberlain and, ultimately, King in 1979.

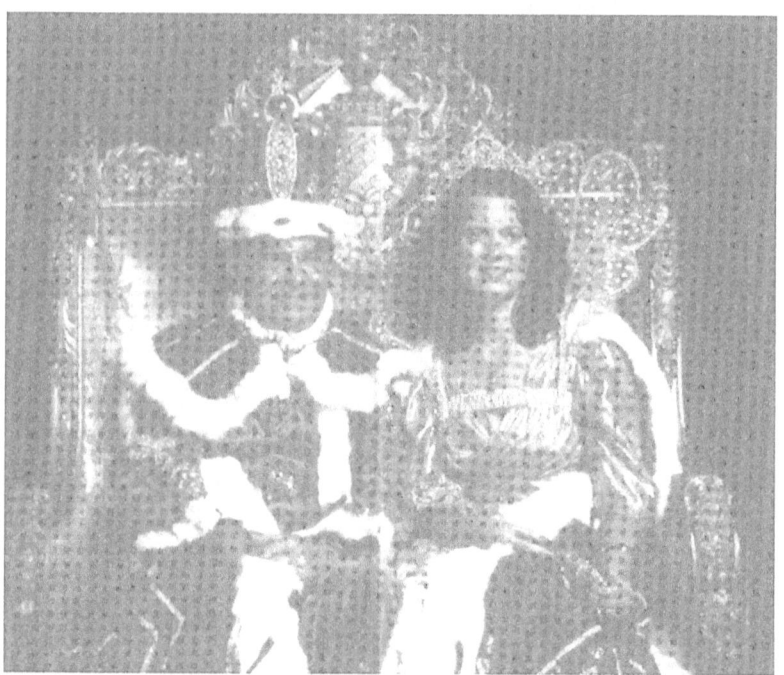

Dr. Ingram as king of Ye Mystic Krewe of Gasparilla, 1979

Having grown up in Florida, Dr. Ingram enjoyed fishing and the beaches and spent a great deal of leisure time in fulfillment of social responsibilities at his beloved home, Journey's End, in Boca Grande, Florida. Much family time was spent there as well. During the annual Gasparilla Pirate Festival as well as other times, he brought to Tampa and Boca Grande many luminaries in the field of OB-GYN, introducing them to the Tampa Bay area.

He took great interest in the history of Tampa and regularly published biographies of local prominent physicians (Ingram 1971, 58:53; Ingram 1978, 65:902) as well as other essays relating to the history of the area (Ingram 1982).

Despite Dr. Ingram's many accomplishments, he always had time to mentor and advise those who came to seek his wisdom, and he always did so in a courtly manner, thus earning him the moniker of Gentleman Jim. In recognition of his character, his personality, and medical acumen, there are two endowed chairs in his name, one at Duke University: the James M. Ingram Professorship of Gynecologic Oncology (established in 1982) and the second, the James M. Ingram Professorship of Obstetrics and Gynecology at the University of South Florida Morsani College of Medicine (established in 1990).

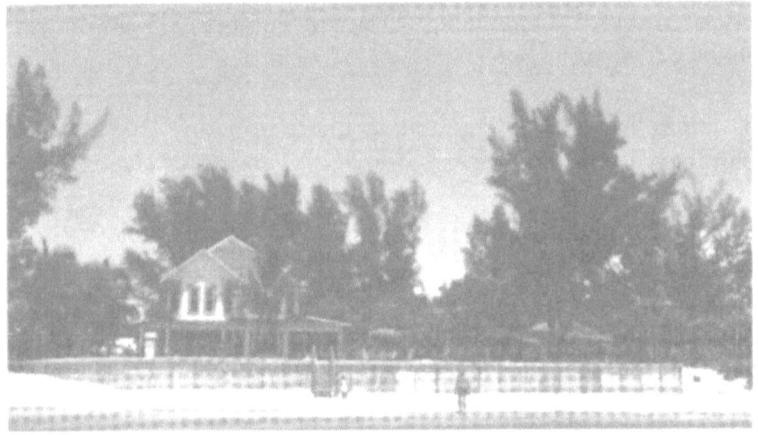

Journey's End in Boca Grande, Florida

While he enjoyed life, always conducting himself in a proper and gentlemanly manner, he never lost sight of his goals and obligations. Taped to the base of the lamp on his desk in the OB-GYN chairman's office at USF was the last stanza of Robert Frost's poem "Stopping by Woods on a Snowy Evening."

> *The woods are lovely, dark and deep,*
> *But I have promises to keep,*
> *And miles to go before I sleep,*
> *And miles to go before I sleep.*

References

Ingram, James M., and Emil Novak. 1951. "Endometrial Carcinoma Associated With Feminizing Ovarian Tumors." *American Journal of Obstetrics & Gynecology.*

Ingram, James M. 1972. "Suprapubic Cystotomy by Trocar Catheter: A Preliminary Report." *American Journal of Obstetrics & Gynecology.*

Sharpe, John R., and James M. Ingram. 1973. "Suprapubic Cystotomy by Trocar Catheter." *Journal of Urology.*

McIndoe, A. 1938. "The Treatment of Congenital Absence and Obliteration Conditions of the Vagina." *Journal of Obstetrics and Gynaecology of the British Commonwealth.*

Wharton, L. R. 1938. "Simple Method of Constructing a Vagina: A Report of Four Cases." *Annals of Surgery.*

Abbe, R. 1898. "New Method of Creating a Vagina in a Case of Congenital Absence." NY Med. Rec.

Frank, R. T. 1938. "The Formation of an Artificial Vagina Without Operation." *American Journal of Obstetrics & Gynecology.*

Ingram, James M. 1981. "The Bicycle Seat Stool in the Treatment of Vaginal Agenesis and Stenosis: A Preliminary Report." *American Journal of Obstetrics & Gynecology.*

Ingram, James M. 1971. "Dr. Louis Simms Oppenheimer: Culture Among the Sandspurs." *Journal of the Florida Medical Association.*

Ingram, James M. 1978. "Some Personal Recollections of Coy Lay." *Journal of the Florida Medical Association.*

Ingram, James M. 1982. "Some Historical and Descriptive Notes on Ye Mystic Krewe of Gasparilla." *The Bulletin* of Hillsborough County Medical Association.

Table 1

USF Medical Students Entering Obstetrics and Gynecology as a Specialty

Year 1974–2010	Total Graduates	Number of Graduates OB-GYN	Percentage of Graduates Who Entered OB-GYN
1974	23	3	13%
1975	25	1	4%
1976	32	2	6.25%
1977	64	5	7.80%
1978	67	7	10.40%
1979	95	10	10.50%
1980	96	12	12.50%
1981	93	7	7.50%
1982	89	7	7.80%
1983	8	0	0%
1984	92	6	6.50%
1985	90	6	6.60%
1986	91	7	7.60%
1987	92	10	10.80%
1988	91	5	5.40%
1989	93	7	7.50%
1990	93	9	9.60%
1991	86	5	5.80%
1992	89	6	6.70%
1993	96	8	8.30%
1994	92	8	8.60%
1995	96	7	7.20%
1996	86	5	5.80%
1997	89	5	5.60%
1998	94	3	3.10%
1999	90	14	15.50%
2000	93	4	4.30%
2001	90	5	5.50%
2002	104	4	3.80%
2003	97	9	9.20%
2004	89	3	3.30%
2005	103	5	4.80%
2006	93	3	3.20%
2007	116	8	6.80%
2008	115	4	3.40%
2009	115	6	5.20%
2010	121	10	8.20%
Total	3,180	266	7.10%

Table 2

Residents Serving Under James M. Ingram Jr., MD

Year	Resident	Medical School	Fac./Fell.
1971–72	Fernando Dolenz, MD		
1972–73	Clifford Levitt, MD	Temple University	
1973–74	James Bassinger, MD	University of Arkansas	
1974–75	Larry Capps, MD	University of South Carolina	
	Larry DeAngelo, MD	Emory University	
	Glen Moore, MD	University of Kentucky	
1975–76	Marguerita Gelpi, MD	University of Miami	
	James Goodrich, MD	Wayne State University	
	Armando Nicholas Gutierrez, MD	University of Miami	
1976–77	Jay J. Garcia, MD	Temple University	
	Frederick Kurtzman, MD	Univ. of the Sciences, Phila.	
1977–78	Rufus (Randy) Armstrong, MD	University of South Florida	
	Wayne S. Blocker, MD	University of Miami	
	Margaret L. Struthers, MD	University of South Florida	
1978–79	William David Gilmer, MD		
	Arthur Perkins, MD	University of Florida	
1979–80	Jack Copeland, MD	Saint Louis University	
	John Herbert, MD		
	Galen Jones, MD	University of South Florida	
	Ruth Petrucha, MD	University of Florida	
1980–81	Eunice Louise Johnson, MD	University of Kentucky	
	Cheryl Bowman Mann, MD	University of South Florida	
	Luciano A. Martinez, MD	University of South Florida	
	Michael T. McNamara, MD	University of Vermont	
1981–82	Robert Clayton, MD	University of South Florida	
	Gregory Eads, MD	West Virginia Univ. SOM	

	Lee Hambrick, MD	Medical College of Georgia	
	Deborah Trehy, MD	University of South Florida	
1982–83	Pam Padillia, MD	University of South Florida	
	Cora Salvino, MD	Chicago Medical School	
	James Von Thron, MD	University of South Florida	
	Ted Von Zeilenski, MD	University of Virginia	
1983–84	Jeffrey Angel, MD	University of South Florida	M/F
	John Cohee, MD	University of Miami	
	Kathleen Kilbride, MD	University of South Florida	
	Buck Mann, MD	University of South Florida	
	Greg Wilkerson, MD	University of Miami	
1984–85	Darryl Ayers, MD		
	Mitchel Hoffman, MD	University of South Florida	O/F
	Brian McNulty, MD	University of South Florida	
	William Newton, MD	University of South Florida	
	George Toskey, MD	Wake Forest University	
1985–86	Kyle Crofoot, MD	University of South Florida	
	James Fiorica, MD	Tufts University	O/F
	Michael Lewis, MD	University of South Florida	
	Jack Lucas, MD	University of North Carolina	
	Valerie Mechanik, MD	University of South Florida	
1986–87	William Brown, MD		
	David O'Bryan, MD	Louisiana State University	
	Frank Marsilisi, MD	Mich. St. Col. of Human Med.	
	Sharon Smith, MD	University of Tennessee	
	Melinda Warren Michelson, MD	East Carolina University	
1987–88	Michael Finazzo, MD	University of Miami	
	Susan Gaylord, MD	Medical College of Penn.	
	Lloyd Lewis, MD	Indiana University	
	Jeff Marks, MD	Case Western Reserve	
	Jeff Michelson, MD	University of South Florida	

Fellowships

M—Maternal-Fetal Medicine
O—Oncology
R—Reproductive Endocrinology and Infertility
U—Urogynecology

F—Faculty

Table 3

Faculty under James M. Ingram Jr., MD*

Anthony Messina, MD
Barry S. Verkauf, MD
Charles Hochberg, MD
Denis Cavanagh, MD
George Maroulis, MD
Greg Wilkerson, MD
Hora Praphat, MD
J. K. Williams, MD
James Goodrich, MD
Jeff Angel, MD
Jose Scerbo, MD
Pierre Bouis, MD
Robert Knupple, MD
Robert Vermillion, MD
Steven Welden, MD
William O'Brien, MD
William Roberts, MD

---

* *Arranged in alphabetical order by first name.*

Table 4

Publications, Peer-Review Journals, and Book Chapters by James M. Ingram, MD*

Journals

1. Ingram, James M., and Emil Novak. "Endometrial Carcinoma Associated with Feminizing Ovarian Tumors." *American Journal of Obstetrics & Gynecology* 61 (April 1951): 774.
2. Ingram, James M., Robert L. Alter, and Bayard Carter. "Occult Rupture of the Uterus." *American Journal of Obstetrics & Gynecology* 64 (September 192): 327.
3. Ingram, James M., Robert W. Withers, and Henry L. Wright. "Vaginal Hysterectomy after Previous Pelvic Surgery." *American Journal of Obstetrics & Gynecology* 74, no 6 (December 1957): 1181.
4. Ingram, James M., Robert W. Withers, and Henry L. Wright. "The Debated Indications for Vaginal Hysterectomy." *Southern Medical Journal* 51, no 7 (July 1958): 869.
5. Ingram, James M. "Pyophysometra Exceeding One Gallon." *American Journal of Obstetrics & Gynecology* 84 (October 1962): 852.
6. Ingram, James M. "Maternal Death in Florida." *Journal of the Florida Medical Association* 50 (November 1962): 415.
7. Ingram, James M. "Maternal Death in Florida." *Journal of the Florida Medical Association* 51 (March 1964): 178.
8. Ingram, James M. "Maternal Death in Florida." *Journal of the Florida Medical Association* 52 (March 1965): 197.
9. Ingram, James M. "Dr. John P. Wall: A Man for All Seasons." A biography in the *Journal of the Florida Medical Association* 53 (August 1966): 8.
10. Ingram, James M., H. S. B. Treloar, G. Phillips Thomas, and Edward B. Road. "Interruption of Pregnancy of Psychiatric Indication: A Suggested Method of Control." *Obstetrics & Gynecology* 29, no 2 (1967): 251.
11. Ingram, James M. "Dr. Howell Tyson Lykes Founder of An Empire (biography)." *Journal of the Florida Medical Association* 55 (August 1968): 742.
12. Ingram, James M. "Changing Aspects of Abortion Law." *American Journal of Obstetrics & Gynecology* 105, no 1 (September 1969): 35.

* *As listed in curriculum vitae*

13. Ingram, James M. "Dr. Louis Simms Oppenheimer: Culture Among the Sandspurs (biography)." *Journal of the Florida Medical Association* 58, no 8 (August 1971): 53.

14. Ingram, James M. "Suprapubic Cystotomy by Trocar Catheter: A Preliminary Report." American Journal of Obstetrics & Gynecology 113 (1972): 1108.

15. Sharp, John R., and James M. Ingram. "Suprapubic Cystostomy by Trocar Catheter." *The Journal of Urology* 110 (September 1973): 340.

16. Levitt, Clifford A., and James M. Ingram. "Abdominal Pregnancy with Complete Ureteral Obstruction: A Case Report." *American Journal of Obstetrics & Gynecology* 120, no2 (September 1974): 3–204.

17. Ingram, James M. "Further Experience with Suprapubic Drainage by Trocar Catheter." *American Journal of Obstetrics & Gynecology* 121, no 7 (April 1975): 885–891.

18. Ingram, James M. "The Presidential Address: A Rebuttal and a Defense." *American Journal of Obstetrics & Gynecology* 123, no 1 (September 1975): 1–5.

19. Ingram, James M. "Some Personal Recollections of Coy Lay." *Fertility and Sterility* 29, no 6 (June 1978): 604.

20. Garcia, Jay J., Barry S. Verkauf, Charles J. Hochberg, and James M. Ingram. "Aberrant Breast Tissue of the Vulva." *Obstetrics & Gynecology* 52, no 2 (August 1978): 225–2228.

21. Ingram, James M. "Some Personal Recollections of Coy Lay." *Journal of the Florida Medical Association* 65 (November 1978): 902–3.

22. Cavanagh, D., H. Praphat, J. M. Ingram, W. R. Anderson, and J. H. Shepherd. "The Management of Invasive Carcinoma of the Vulva." *Proceedings of the IX World Congress of Gynecology and Obstetrics*. Amsterdam, The Netherlands, 1980. Excerpta Medica.

23. Ingram, James M. "The Art of Medicine." *Editorial Journal of the Florida Medical Association* 68 (January 1981): 10–11.

24. Ingram, James M. "The Bicycle Seat Stool in the Treatment of Vaginal Agenesis and Stenosis: A Preliminary Report." *American Journal of Obstetrics & Gynecology* 140, no 8 (August 1981): 867–873.

25. Ingram, James. M. "The Change of Life at 50." *Journal of the Florida Medical Association* 68 (September 1981): 758.

Chapters

1. "Postoperative Bladder Drainage." In *Gynecologic and Obstetric Urology*, edited by Buchsbaum and Schmidt. W.B. Saunders Co., 1977.
2. "Endometriosis." In *Current Obstetrics and Gynecologic Diagnosis and Treatment*, edited by Benson. Lange Medical Publications, 1978, 1980, 1982, 1984.
3. "Pelvic Inflammatory Disease." In *Current Therapy in Obstetrics & Gynecology*, edited by Quilligan. W.B. Saunders Co., 1980.
4. "Vulvovaginitis and Cervicitis." In *Precis*, edited by American Congress of Obstetricians and Gynecologists. Second ed. McGraw and Hill, 1982.
5. "Postoperative Management of the Bladder." In *Gynecology and Obstetrics*, edited by J. J. Sciarra. Harper & Row Publishers, 1984.
6. "Vulvar Dystrophy." In *Current Therapy in Obstetrics & Gynecology*, edited by Quilligan and Zuspan. Third ed. W.B. Saunders Co., 1989.

Historical Publications

1. Ingram, James M. "Journey's End: The History of an Island Home." First ed. Florida: Hillsborough Press, 1962. Reprinted 1963 with second edition 1980.
2. Ingram, James M. "Henry B. Plant., Dr. Louis Oppenheimer, and the Tampa Bay Hotel." *The Bulletin* of the Hillsborough County Medical Association. (November 1980, December 1980).
3. Ingram, James M. "Some Historical and Descriptive Notes on Ye Mystic Krewe of Gasparilla." *The Bulletin* of the Hillsborough County Medical Association (February 1982).
4. Ingram, James M. "St. Joseph's Hospital: The First 50 years." *The Bulletin* of the Hillsborough County Medical Association (September 1984).
5. Ingram, James M. "Demographic Changes in Medical Practice in Tampa, 1951–1986." *The Bulletin* of the Hillsborough County Medical Association (January 1987).

Exhibits

1. Ingram, James M. Biographic sketches and memorabilia of various physicians for whom the OB-GYN wards at Duke Medical Center were named. Displayed on the wards since 1950.

CHAPTER 2

Evolution of the Department of Obstetrics and Gynecology

by *Barry S. Verkauf, MD, MBA*

In 1963, President John F. Kennedy signed a bill providing over three billion dollars for expansion of medical services, medical schools, medical education, and facilities to improve the health of Americans. This was apparently in response to the low number of physicians in the country compared to the future health needs of the country. Much of this money was distributed in the form of matching grants whereby local facilities would provide one-third of the money and the federal government would match this two dollars to one. Many of these schools were formed in conjunction with an increasing number of Veterans Health Administration hospitals to be made available for a growing number of aged veterans after the First and Second World Wars and the Korean War.

The Early Years

This availability of funds stimulated the interest of the citizens of the Tampa area to have a medical school. This was fueled by the fact that, at the time, Florida was one of the fastest-growing states and the Tampa Bay area was one of the fastest-growing areas within it. Moreover, Tampa, centrally located in the state, was without a school of medicine although one already existed in the north-central area of the state (at the University of Florida) and another in the southern part of the state (at the University of Miami).

Congressman Sam Gibbons was instrumental in making appropriate contacts locally and in Washington, DC, to encourage interest in Tampa. The lead locally was initiated by physicians in the community, organized within the Hillsborough County Medical Association under the auspices of a committee on the medical school reporting to the board of directors of the HCMA. The initial committee on the medical school included Drs. Richard Connar, Louis Cimino, Joseph Flynn, H. Phillip Hampton, Samuel G. Hibbs, James M. Ingram, Lawrence Kahana, Sorrell Wolfson, and Robert W. Withers.

While freestanding community residencies already existed at Tampa General Hospital, the appeal of this form of residency training was diminishing compared to that affiliated with an academic institution. These were the driving forces for bringing a college of medicine to a community that already had good medical care and community residency-education programs.

While initial thoughts were that this college of medicine might be an outreach from the University of Florida but located in metropolitan Tampa, the University of South Florida, having opened with its first class of students in 1960, became a more natural allied entity. The University of South Florida and its first president, Dr. James Allen, were interested in incorporating a college of medicine within the university and encouraged the committee of physicians already formed by the HCMA to spearhead this effort.

On the committee for medical schools from its inception (and its chairman in 1968 prior to becoming president of the HCMA in 1969) was James M. Ingram, MD. His partners in practice at the time, Dr. Robert Withers and Dr. Henry Wright, were also instrumental in pushing efforts for the medical school.

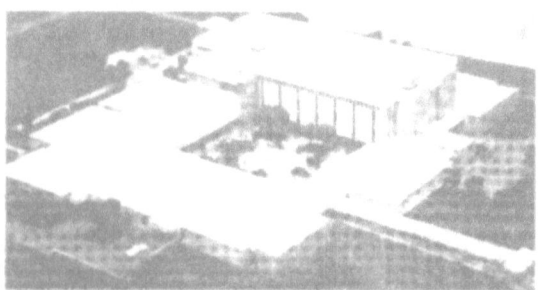

Initial structures at the new USF medical school

Of course, there were many bumps in the road along the way relative to state support, follow-through of government funding, and interpolitical squabbles, but the first permanent dean of the medical school—Donn L. Smith, PhD—was appointed in 1969, and plans were rapidly made for development of a medical school in three phases: The first, related to the basic sciences, a library and basic science faculty offices; the second, related to growth of clinical departments, faculty offices, enlargement of the library, a cafeteria, some research facilities, a clinical facility for faculty to see patients, and a medical auditorium; and the third phase, which was given some consideration but ultimately decided against, was a university hospital of three hundred beds—the need for which was questioned since Florida Hospital Tampa existed across the street from the medical school and because of the availability of the 720-bed James A. Haley Veterans' Hospital, planned and under construction, along with Tampa General Hospital's already existing engagement in medical education and availability for medical school and resident teaching. The first affiliation agreement between USF and TGH was in 1970, under which Dr. Jack Hickman was the first director of medical education.

The principal charge of the new medical school was to educate physicians for clinical practice to serve Florida communities. Interdigitation between faculty and the medical community was to have been significant, and there was a desire for town-gown relationships to be good. Many members of the practicing medical community in Tampa were involved in the planning of the medical school, providing sweat equity, and emotional or other support, and exceeded fifty in number. Among the most prominent of these was James Ingram. Dr. Ingram was one of the first five clinical faculty members to be appointed at the medical school, serving as the first professor and chairman of the Department of Obstetrics and Gynecology beginning in 1970. He was present when the first class of medical students matriculated in the new school in 1971–72, and by the school year of 1972–73, when the first class of students entered their clinical years, twelve of forty-eight academic appointments in the college of medicine were within the Department of Obstetrics and Gynecology. In addition to Dr. Ingram, the eleven other appointments were at the voluntary clinical level among interested clinicians in the obstetric and gynecologic community, including Drs. Albert Cohen, Richard Crane, Joseph Levine, Byrne Marston, Robert McCammon, Byron Metts, Jack Mezrah, Harold Nix, James Phillips, Robert Qualey, and G. Phillips Thomas. Dr. Ingram took to heart the need to integrate the medical community into the medical school's activities at its onset to ensure its success, and he served as a liaison and buffer between the community and the academic environment. The number of volunteers for the clinical faculty always exceeded the number required, and these were rotated on a yearly basis.

Changing Times

The Department of Obstetrics and Gynecology was the first clinically oriented academic department up and running at the newly formed medical school. At the outset, Dr. Coy Lay from Lakeland volunteered as part-time faculty to drive over each week and spend Friday mornings teaching the medical students and residents. Dr. Lay was a unique man. His training had taken place contemporaneously with Dr. Ingram, but at the Mayo Clinic. He always had an interest in maintaining scholarly relationships with well-trained obstetrician-gynecologists around the country, and he did so principally by starting the *Collected Letters in Obstetrics and Gynecology*, which he edited, and regularly asked prominent clinicians around the country to write answers to questions he posed or that were sent in by doctors who subscribed to the letter. Moreover, he was a founding partner of the Watson Clinic in Lakeland, a prominent multispecialty clinic, but most importantly, because of his interest in infertility and endoscopy, ultimately became president (in 1975) of what at the time was called The American Fertility Society (now the American Society for Reproductive Medicine). Playboy magazine had a good time with this set of circumstances, drawing attention in one of their issues to the fact that "the new President of The American Fertility Society is Dr. Coy Lay!"

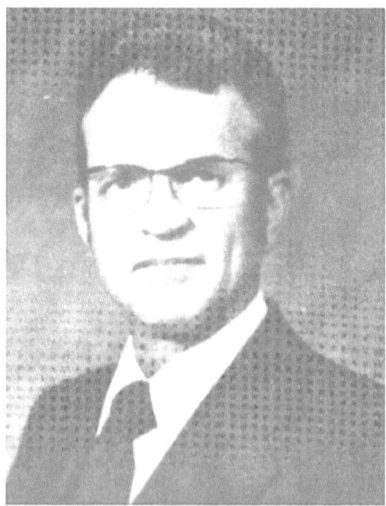

Dr. Coy L. Lay

Dr. Lay was an excellent endoscopist and a personal friend of Patrick Steptoe, the internationally renowned endoscopist from England, who worked with Robert Edwards in achieving the first in-vitro-fertilization birth in 1978. Dr. Lay devised a method of occluding the fallopian tubes through a laparoscope. At that time, there was an emphasis on contraceptive methods, and new techniques were quite fashionable.

While Dr. Ingram had eleven clinical assistant professors appointed from the community to aid in imparting knowledge to the up-and-coming first class of medical students, all these men were generalists in obstetrics and gynecology, as was Dr. Ingram. But Dr. Ingram recognized the tides of change that were swirling about in the academic OB-GYN community. With increasing federal research support and increasing breadth and depth of knowledge within the field of OB-GYN, there was much discussion about the need for evolution of subspecialties within obstetrics and gynecology, like those already existing in internal medicine (e.g., nephrology, cardiology, gastroenterology, and the like).

Three subspecialty areas were envisioned within obstetrics and gynecology: reproductive endocrinology and infertility, gynecologic oncology, and maternal-fetal medicine. Dr. Ingram was able to appreciate the inevitability of increasing specialization and the need to supplement his faculty with young, full-time members with interest and expertise in these areas. In 1972, official boards were formed to certify these subspecialists although the first certifying exams were not offered until 1974.

The second full-time faculty member in the department was Dr. Charles Hochberg, who came to the University of South Florida right out of residency at the University of Rochester where he developed an interest in maternal-fetal medicine under the tutelage of Dr. Curtis Lund and Dr. Mortimer Rosen. Dr. Hochberg took on the principal responsibility of teaching residents and students complicated obstetrics. He was an energetic, optimistic, affable young man, well liked by everyone. Based on his experience at Rochester, Dr. Hochberg instituted the tradition of Resident's Day at which all residents presented scientific papers during June of each year, a tradition that continues within the department to this day. He was an excellent supplement to Dr. Ingram, whose history of community involvement and intimate knowledge of the Tampa community bridged the gap between "town and gown." This good relationship between the town and the university remained throughout Dr. Ingram's tenure as professor and chairman.

Dr. Barry Verkauf joined the department in 1974 as the third full-time faculty member. Dr. Verkauf came to the University of South Florida after having completed two years in the military subsequent to serving as chief resident in the six-year OB-GYN residency program at Johns Hopkins Hospital. While there, he received training under the auspices of prominent physicians Drs. Howard and Georgeanna Jones. Dr. Georgeanna Jones was the first reproductive endocrinologist in the United States and initiated the first division of reproductive endocrinology and infertility in the United States at Hopkins. Dr. Howard Jones was a gynecologic surgeon with a particular interest in congenital anomalies, surgical infertility, and the new discipline of genetics, offering Dr. Verkauf a comprehensive exposure to this field during his residency experience and a fellowship spent with the Joneses. Dr. Verkauf was charged with student and resident teaching in the area of reproductive endocrinology and infertility within the department. He also had the responsibility of developing postgraduate-education programs for the department.

During this period of time, resident clinics for patients without insurance were in existence at Tampa General Hospital in all specialties for which there were residency programs. Dr. Verkauf initiated a reproductive endocrine and infertility clinic at Tampa General and guided residents and students in that clinic for many years.

Also in 1974, Dr. Robert Vermillion joined the department, having completed his residency at the Johns Hopkins Hospital as well. Dr. Vermillion's interests were principally in gynecologic surgery and endoscopy. The Yoon band had been developed at Hopkins as an occlusive device for tubal sterilization through the endoscope, and there were many "friendly" discussions between Dr. Lay and Dr. Vermillion about whose technique was best!

Dr. Vermillion also had the responsibility within the department of overseeing the teaching program for medical students. At that time, medical students at USF were on a three-year program. They had two weeks off at Christmas and two weeks off in the summer but, otherwise, were in class year-round. Despite this somewhat shortened academic experience for USF medical students in these early years, they regularly scored highly on their local and national exams relative to the topics of obstetrics and gynecology, and a high proportion of students from USF entered the field of obstetrics and gynecology.

Learning to perform a clinical pelvic exam has always been difficult for students and residents. Feedback from the patient, particularly if they are ill, is often hard to interpret, and having healthy women give feedback on the correctness of performing the pelvic exam seemed of obvious value. Dr. Vermillion established the second program in the country, hiring paid volunteers whom medical students and residents were able to perform pelvic exams on and getting intelligent, appropriate feedback from these volunteers, thus enabling young doctors to learn how to perform pelvic exams on women with greater skill.

Dr. Vermillion also had the responsibility for teaching medical students and residents gynecologic pathology as he had academic strength in this area, having trained at Hopkins—the birthplace of gynecologic pathology—under Dr. Emil Novak and, subsequently, Dr. J. Donald Woodruff. Dr. Vermillion's efforts were critical in imparting the important clinicopathological correlation in treating gynecologic diseases. He complemented the efforts of Dr. Eugene Ruffolo of the Pathology Department at TGH in this regard. Dr. Ruffolo was board-certified in both obstetrics and gynecology and pathology and spent many hours contributing his knowledge on a voluntary basis to USF medical students and OB-GYN residents.

In 1975, Dr. Anthony M. Messina came from the University of Florida, having completed his residency, to join the young cadre of new full-time faculty members. Dr. Messina's interests were always in gynecologic surgery and gynecologic oncology. He was a skilled and well-educated physician who found the department with young, industrious, and well-educated faculty members a titillating and informative environment. Over the ensuing years, Dr. Messina had much interaction in teaching the medical students and operating with the residents. He took pride in emphasizing the comprehensive precepts necessary to become a "good doctor." These efforts were often expressed by and were well appreciated by the residents exposed to him.

The academic offices for the department were in the old Gordon Keller Nursing School Building (now the site of the parking garage) adjacent to Tampa General Hospital. Dot Place and Betty Monti were the two secretaries for all five members of the department.

To maintain and refine their clinical skills, the University Medical Service Association (UMSA) had been formed for all clinical-faculty members to have an organizational structure within which they could see private patients. The private offices of the Department of Obstetrics and Gynecology were housed in One Davis Boulevard, a building preexisting the medical school by over a decade and that still stands today across the street from Tampa General Hospital. Most of the inpatient clinical activities of the full-time Department of Obstetrics and Gynecology were carried out at Tampa General Hospital, though occasional obstetrical deliveries were made at St. Joseph's Hospital.

In 1976, the medical clinics on the University of South Florida campus, part of the second phase of development of the medical school, were completed. Dr. Ingram began seeing his private patients in that facility and, in fact, had the distinction of serving the first patient ever seen within

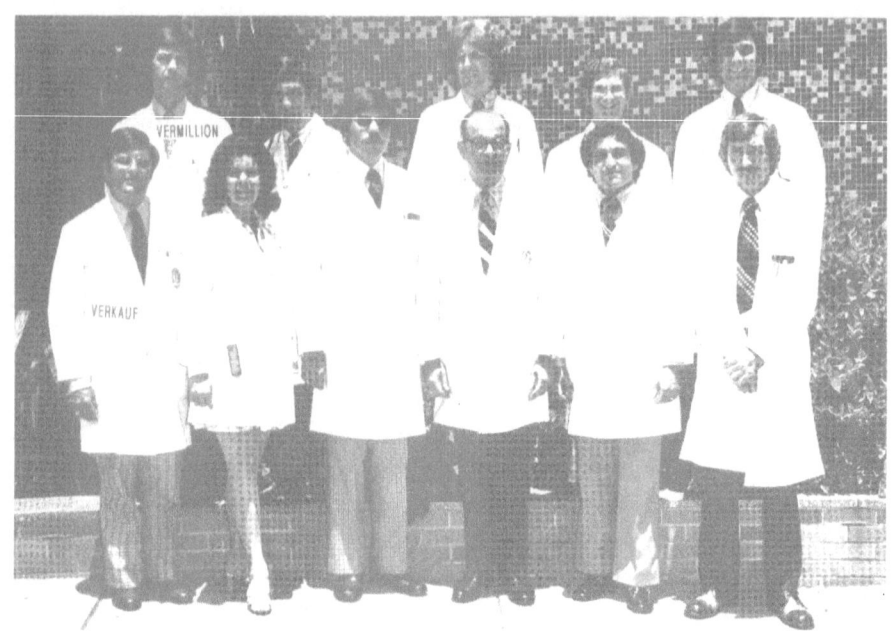

Dr. Barry S. Verkauf and Dr. Robert Vermillion with residents, 1975

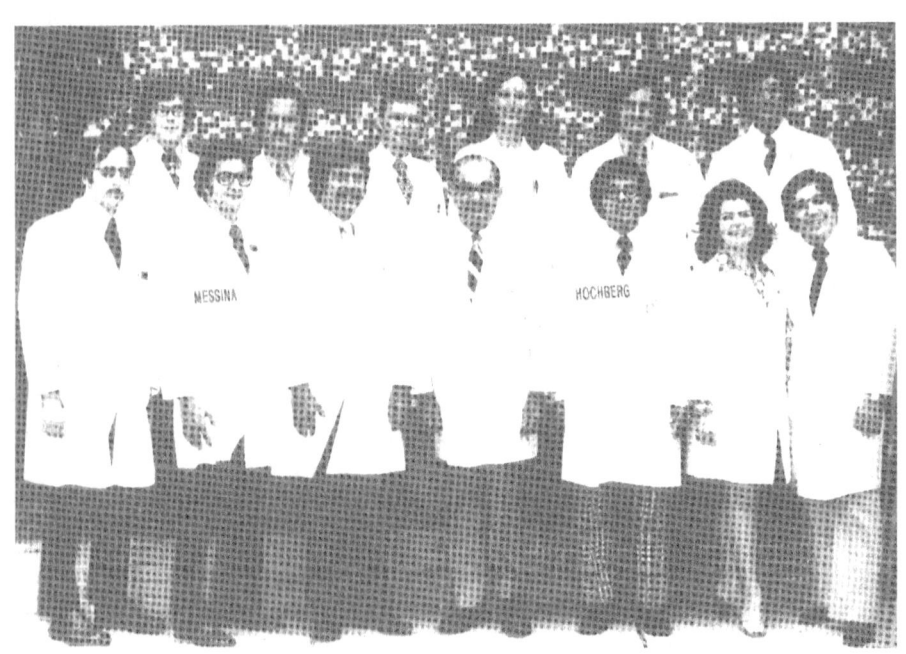

Dr. Charles Hochberg and Dr. Anthony Messina with residents, 1976

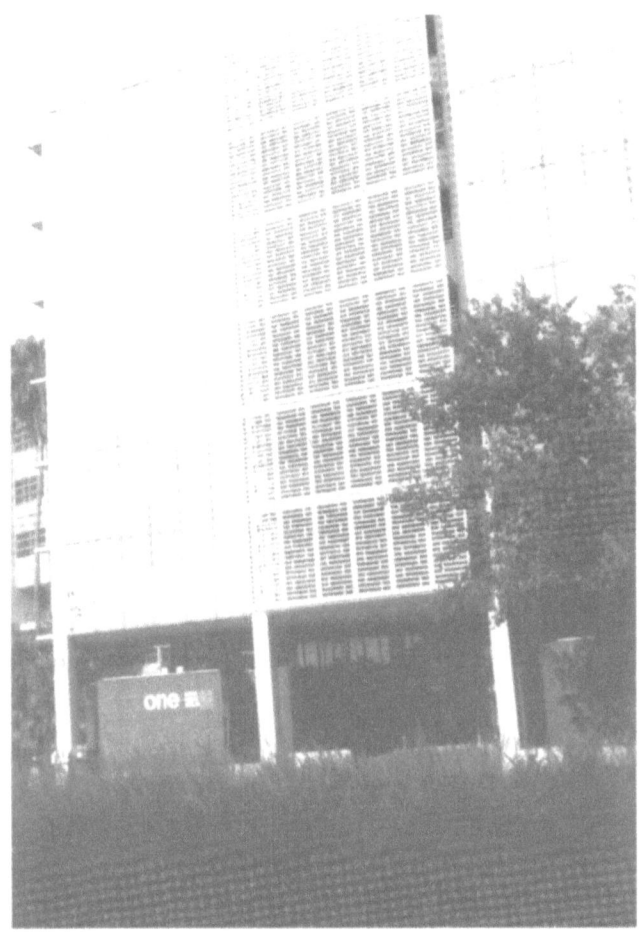

One Davis Boulevard office building, earliest offices of University Medical Services Association at University of South Florida Morsani College of Medicine

that new facility. Subsequently, Dr. James Goodrich established an ongoing gynecology clinic at the James A. Haley Veterans' Hospital.

In 1977, Dr. Pierre Bouis joined the faculty, having completed his medical school and residency education at the Louisiana State University. Dr. Bouis was trained in both obstetrics and gynecology and in radiology. He also had interest in graduate medical education and after leaving for a brief stint in private practice, returned to the department in 1978 with a joint appointment in obstetrics and gynecology and as assistant dean in continuing medical education.

An unanticipated, fortunate addition to the faculty in 1978 was Dr. Denis Cavanagh. Unlike those members of the full-time faculty already present, all of whom were young and entered faculty positions just out of residency training or military service, Dr. Cavanagh was older, an experienced as well as highly renowned figure within obstetrics and gynecology. Although he had many clinical interests, Dr. Cavanagh's specialty was gynecologic oncology. He had previously served on the faculty at the University of Miami and had been professor and chairman of obstetrics and gynecology at the Saint Louis University School of Medicine and at the University of Tasmania in Australia. With Dr. Cavanagh from Saint Louis, as an associate professor came Dr. Hora Praphat and also Papeneia Rao, PhD. Dr. Praphat, like Dr. Cavanagh, was a skilled and experienced surgeon in gynecologic oncology, and Dr. Rao was the first full-time research PhD within the department. This was the beginning of the evolution of a structured division of gynecologic oncology and a division with both bench and clinical research within it. A fellowship in gynecologic oncology was quickly established. Dr. William Roberts joined the faculty as assistant professor in 1982, and a yearly train of excellent national and international fellows followed. During the early years of the department, before Dr. Cavanagh's arrival, Dr. Harold Sanders, in private practice in Tampa and a skilled oncologic surgeon trained at Sloan-Kettering, often scrubbed with residents on gynecologic oncologic procedures.

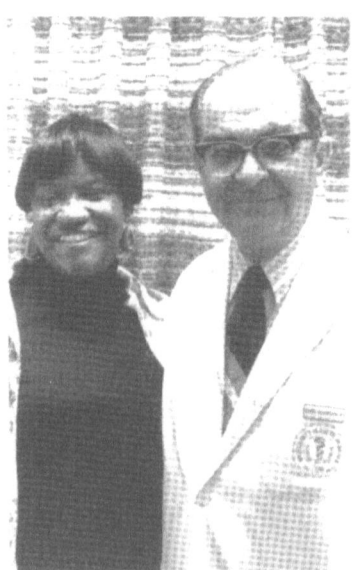

Dr. Ingram with the first patient seen at the new medical clinic facility on campus of the USF Morsani Medical School, 1976

One year later, Dr. Robert Knuppel joined the faculty. Dr. Knuppel was board-certified in maternal fetal medicine, having completed his fellowship and two years on the faculty at Tufts University. He was joined shortly thereafter by Dr. Jose Scerbo and began structuring a formal division of maternal fetal medicine with a board-approved fellowship soon filled with a long line of promising maternal fetal medicine fellows. Dr. J. K. Williams was recruited from Wayne State University in 1982 as assistant professor and director of the residency program and was later joined by Dr. Steven Welden from the University of Tennessee as director of the student clerkship.

As is common, as new members joined the faculty, some earlier members left for other opportunities, but the growth of the department and its responsibilities to an increasing number of residents and students continued. The original medical-school class size of twenty-eight students had, by 1975, grown to ninety students, and the number of residents accepted per year for training had increased from three to four. Agreements were made in 1976 with the Ruskin County Migrant Health Center for greater patient access for students, residents, and fellows. Moreover, a relationship was established with the community OB-GYN residency at Bayfront Health in Saint Petersburg in 1976 and with St. Joseph's Women's Hospital in Tampa—the latter, a private hospital where residents had the opportunity to be involved in the care of private patients under the direction of community physicians. The Bayfront residency was under the direction of Dr. Richard Anderson and, subsequently, Dr. Charles McCurdy. A committee on education was formed at St. Joseph's Women's Hospital to oversee resident activities there. Community physicians from Pinellas County and Hillsborough County continued to play important roles and made significant contributions to student and residency teaching. Moreover, from surrounding counties, academically oriented physicians—such as Dr. Tim Howell from Winter Haven and Dr. Vincent Stenger from Sarasota—volunteered their time and efforts.

CHAPTER 3

Midwinter Seminar in Obstetrics and Gynecology

by Barry S. Verkauf, MD, MBA

Subsequent to World War II, the innovative techniques and experiences brought back by physicians from these war zones increased governmental support in medical education and new technological advances led to an explosion in knowledge within the field of medicine. The rapidity of change increased, and it was no longer possible for the practicing physician to utilize only the body of knowledge learned in medical school and residency, supplemental reading, and his own personal experience to provide optimum patient care.

Continuing medical education became a watchword during the 1970s when many states passed laws requiring physicians to have a minimum number of hours of continuing medical education, usually in three-year cycles, to supplement their basic knowledge and to ensure up-to-date understanding of the progress in medicine, which could then be incorporated into their clinical practices.

The American Medical Association and the American Congress of Obstetricians and Gynecologists (ACOG) were particularly interested and active in supporting this concept. ACOG, in addition to putting on several of their own postgraduate courses, had the idea that it might be useful to encourage young medical schools to provide such courses and, in doing so, give exposure to their faculty nationally, interest them in new and novel ideas within the field of medicine, and serve as bases around the country from which courses in obstetrics and gynecology could be offered. The plan was to offer approximately eight new medical schools the opportunity to present these courses with the aid of ACOG in providing some guidance, printing of brochures and other materials, and assuring that no department would suffer an economic loss as a consequence of its involvement. By charging for these courses, there was the opportunity for fledgling departments to earn income to supplement the growth of their department. If the course was profitable, the department kept 75 percent of the earnings, and ACOG, 25 percent. If the course was not profitable, all losses were absorbed by ACOG.

In 1975, ACOG came to Dr. Ingram as chairman of the Department of OB-GYN at USF, one of the new medical schools in the country. They discussed the matter with him. Always easily engaged when presented with a new and good opportunity, Dr. Ingram quickly agreed to the challenge. He asked Dr. Barry Verkauf—who, while at Hopkins, had exposure to the Emil Novak postgraduate course presented yearly by the Department of Obstetrics and Gynecology as a preparatory course for those ready to take their board exams—to guide the evolution of the Midwinter Seminar, put it into practice, and maintain its continuation on an annual basis.

Drs. Verkauf and Ingram collaborated on this project and after some discussion, decided on a time, a format, and a mission for the course. Both were quick to realize that Florida had a competitive advantage in the winter as a site for such a course. For those trapped in northern climates and who wished to escape them, a postgraduate course in Florida represented an excellent opportunity to combine getting out of the cold weather, a family vacation, an opportunity to gain knowledge, and the possibility of writing it off as a business expense. Thus, it was decided that the course would be in the winter, and Dr. Ingram coined the name the Midwinter Seminar in Obstetrics and Gynecology. The South Atlantic Association of Obstetricians and Gynecologists (SAAOG), though their meetings were in various climates, also focused on the ability for members to bring and spend time with their families as part of the educational, social, and political experience. Like SAAOG meetings, it was decided that since the physicians were often up early, the course activities would be from 7:00 a.m. until 1:00 p.m., leaving the opportunity for physicians to spend time with their families in the warmth of the Florida sun in the afternoons.

With the advent of subspecialization, it was felt best to focus on subspecialties to provide new knowledge in these areas, inviting nationally recognized physicians to speak and to supplement their talks with lectures by local faculty. There would be a day of obstetrics and maternal-fetal medicine; a day of reproductive endocrinology, infertility, contraception, and related matters; and a day of general gynecology, gynecologic surgery, and gynecological oncology. Each Midwinter Seminar had a unifying theme throughout. For example, one year might focus on issues related to the impact of infection across the obstetrical, gynecological, and infertility/endocrine landscape. Another year might focus on the role of obesity as a complicating factor across the fields of obstetrics, gynecology, and reproductive endocrinology/infertility.

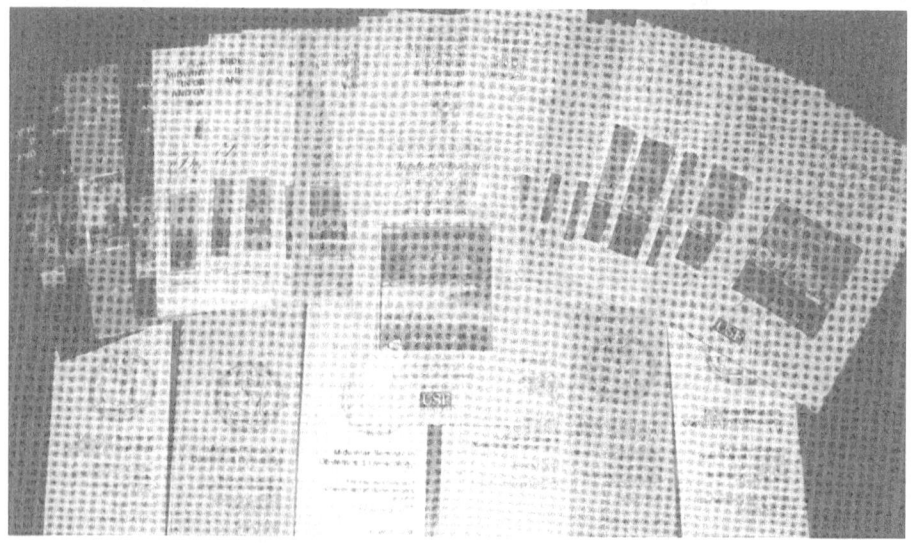

Brochures from multiple Midwinter Seminar programs

The first Midwinter Seminar in Obstetrics and Gynecology took place in February 1976. Because the basic science buildings for the new medical school had just been completed on the University of South Florida campus, it was felt that this should be the venue for the first program, which would be held on a Friday, Saturday, and Sunday. However, weekend construction on the remaining buildings of the medical school had not been anticipated, and the speakers at the Midwinter Seminar had to compete with jackhammers and other construction noises to gain the attention of course attendees. Fortunately, they did so with aplomb.

The first invited guests at the Midwinter Seminar were the nationally known figures Dr. Jack Pritchard, in maternal-fetal medicine, and reproductive endocrinologist Dr. Paul McDonald, both from Parkland Hospital and Southwestern University in Dallas. These were men of unquestioned clinical acumen and academic expertise, and their commitment to fulfilling their responsibilities can be learned from the following unique story:

At the first Midwinter Seminar, subsequent to accepting an invitation to participate, Dr. Paul McDonald received a large grant and donation to fund a chair in his name and further research at his institution. The celebratory event was to be held on the Saturday night during which he was to be in Tampa for the Midwinter. Unbeknownst to Drs. Verkauf and Ingram or any attendees, he gave his discussions on Friday and Saturday, took a plane back to Dallas on Saturday afternoon for the Saturday evening black-tie event, then caught a night flight back to Tampa, arriving in time to complete his scheduled lecture on Sunday regarding the role of prostaglandins in the initiation of labor.

The second Midwinter Seminar in Obstetrics and Gynecology was held in 1977 on the University of South Florida campus in the newly completed medical-school auditorium. While the facilities were excellent for teaching, the logistics of housing attendees was a problem. The University of South Florida had only been in existence for fifteen years, and growth around the university was just beginning to occur. There were only two motels, the best of which was engaged to house participants of the Midwinter Seminar, and it was necessary to arrange buses to transport them each morning from the motel on Fowler Avenue to the classrooms at the university and back to the motel afterward. Moreover, the department being small, there were only two secretaries. With their regular duties, they were unable to attend to the myriad items necessary to put on a well-oiled postgraduate course. Dr. Verkauf turned to women volunteers of the Greater Tampa Chamber of Commerce and to faculty wives to help register guests and facilitate their movement from the motel to the campus and back and to nightly activities in which they were engaged.

While Florida offered many recreational activities for participants at some distance (e.g., Disney World, the beaches), other than Busch Gardens, there were few attractions near the university and essentially no restaurants or activities for nighttime entertainment. Consequently, during the second night of the Midwinter Seminar, all course attendees who wished to attend were taken by bus to a cocktail buffet and dinner at such Tampa classics as the Columbia Restaurant in Ybor City and the University Club downtown. While the auditorium had been built on the main medical-school campus, providing an excellent venue for daytime courses, problems remained with housing guests and making sure that their off time was entertaining and enjoyable. Moreover, the motel facilities limited the number of participants who could be engaged, and after the first year, there were always more registrants than could be accommodated—finally necessitating cutting off attendance at 225 enrollees. All these issues set the need for a different venue, and after a good deal of searching and consideration, Drs. Verkauf and

Ingram decided to move the Midwinter Seminar in 1981 to the Don CeSar Beach Resort Hotel on Saint Petersbug Beach.

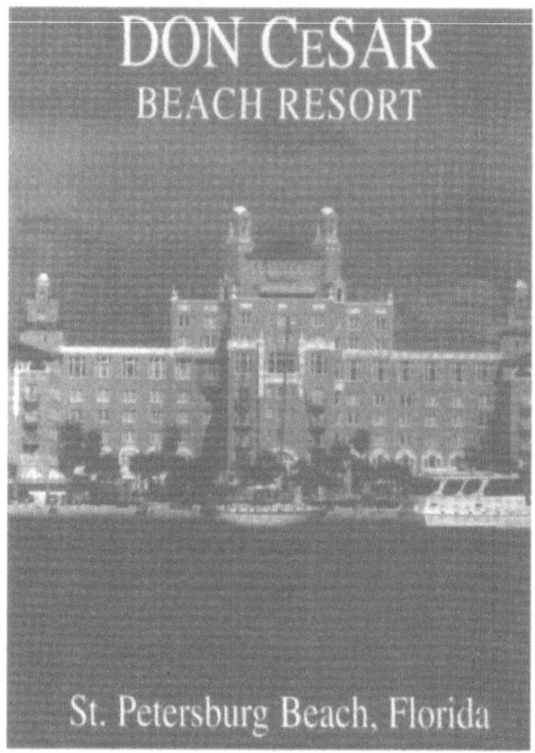

Don CeSar Beach Resort Hotel on Saint Petersburg Beach

This classic Florida resort hotel, built in the boom time of the 1920s, offered an unusual and delightful environment with the availability of the beaches right out the back door and many opportunities for afternoon and evening activity along with Florida's west-coast beach activities on Gulf Boulevard. This proved to be a popular move with course attendees, and the course remained at the Don CeSar for the next two years.

In the early 1980s, Tampa underwent a real-estate boom and new office buildings and hotels were sprouting up in what had been a somewhat tepid downtown. In order to showcase downtown Tampa and take advantage of the publicity associated with the Super Bowl being in Tampa in 1984, the course was moved to the Hyatt Regency Hotel in downtown Tampa. While this proved adequate, course attendees preferred the beach site, and in starting 1985, the beach venue at the Don CeSar was used yearly for the next twenty years. During that interval, with two changes in management and two upgrades in the facility, it remained a delightful and charming vacation spot, as well as one well designed and suitable for the educational format of a 7:00 a.m. to 1:00 p.m. program, which has until recently consistently characterized this postgraduate course.

Many luminaries and important educators in the field of obstetrics and gynecology served as guest speakers at the Midwinter Seminar over its now thirty-five years of existence at this writing. It is one of the longest, consecutive, continuing postgraduate courses in the United States.

Drs. Georgeanna and Howard Jones

This Smile Charmed Patients, Friends, & at least Three Generations of Residents Donald Woodruff, MD.

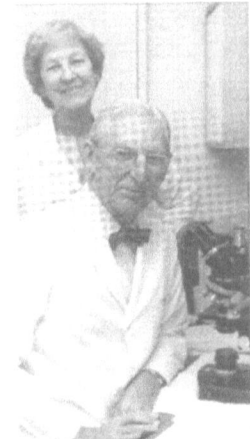
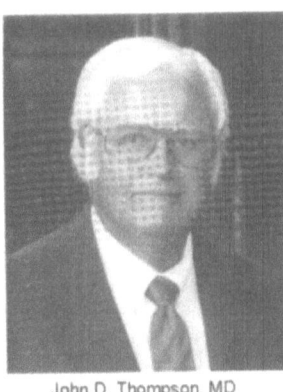
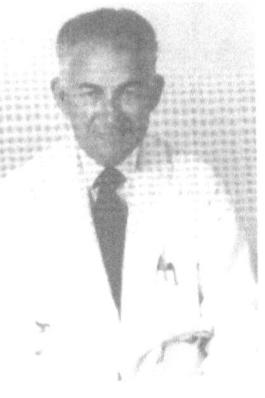

John D. Thompson, MD

Outstanding educators as guest professors at Midwinter Seminar in Obstetrics and Gynecology.

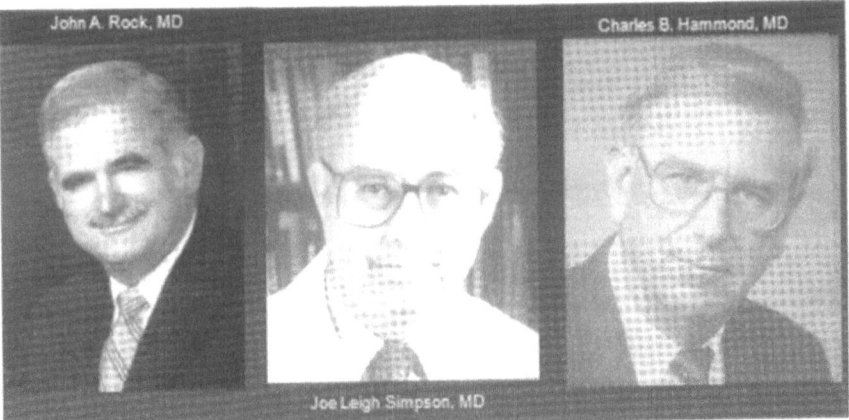

John A. Rock, MD

Charles B. Hammond, MD

Joe Leigh Simpson, MD

Since 2004, Dr. J. K. Williams has assumed directorship of this long-standing and popular postgraduate educational effort. In very recent years, the site of the program, while remaining in a beach environment, has been at the Sheraton Sand Key Resort in Clearwater. Until recently, the course was entirely put on by members of the department and its staff, including the valued help of Cedell McKeever, Candy Smith, Betty Monti, and Dot Place. At present, with the growth of the Office of Professional Development within the university, arrangements for the course are handled by that department, though its direction, content, and structure are determined by the Department of Obstetrics and Gynecology under the direction of Dr. J. K. Williams. The course was renamed the James M. Ingram Midwinter Seminar in Obstetrics and Gynecology following his death in 1989.

Table 5

Guest Faculty Participants in Midwinter Seminar in OB-GYN

Date	Name
1976	Paul McDonald, MD Jack Pritchard, MD Paul Mc Donough, MD
1977	Howard W. Jones Jr., MD Georgeanna Seegar Jones, MD Gerard N. Burrows, MD John Queenan, MD
1978	Taylor Wharton, MD Duane Townsend, MD J. Donald Woodruff, MD Kamran Moghissi, MD
1979	Joe Leigh Simpson, MD Sir John Dewhurst Raymond Kaufman, MD
1980	
1981	Lawrence Kahana, MD Pauline Powers, MD Allen Root, MD Donald Gray, MD
1982	Allen H. DeCherney, MD John D. Thompson, MD John L. Sever, MD Richard Sweet, MD
1983	Robert C. Cefalo, MD, PhD Raymond A. Lee, MD Anne Colston Wentz, MD
1984	Alex A. Bezjian, MD James F. Daniell, MD Donald R. Ostergard, MD Jeffrey A. Shane, MD, JD

1985	Robert Israel, MD Douglas J. Marchant, MD John Marlow, MD
1986	Ricardo Ashe, MD Daniel Mishell, MD Roberto Romero, MD
1987	Charles B. Hammond, MD David H. Nichols, MD William N. Spellacy, MD
1988	John C. Hobbins, MD Roy W. Huntsman, MD Richard P. Marrs, MD
1989	James L. Breen, MD Daniel R. Mishell, MD
1990	Michael Baggish, MD John Marlow, MD David Nichols, MD
1991	Rudolph P. Galask, MD David S. Guzick, MD, PhD Arthur L. Herbst, MD Michael A. Rainey Edward E. Wallach, MD Joan Zinober, PhD, MBA
1992	James Dorsey, MD Arthur Haney, MD Doulas Marchant, MD
1993	Gary Cunningham, MD Howard W. Jones, III, MD Donald Ostergard, MD Zev Rosenwaks, MD
1994	Robert C. Cefalo, MD, PhD Alan H. DeCherney, MD Raymond A. Lee, MD Scott L. Hopes, MPH Joan Zinober, PhD, MBA

1995	Ronald S. Gibbs, MD
	Wayne Heine, MD
	David H. Nichols, MD
	John A. Rock, MD
1996	Robert L. Goldenberg, MD
	William R. Keye Jr., MD
	David L. Olive, MD
	Ralph M. Richard, MD
1997	Mark R. Hughes, MD, PhD
	Charles J. Lockwood, MD
	Paul G. McDonough, MD
	Joseph San Filippo, MD, MBA
1998	Linda Brubaker, MD
	Patrick Duff, MD
	A. Cullen Richardson, MD
	William B. Saye, MD
	Carl P. Weiner, MD
1999	Robert R. Goldenberg, MD
	David L. Olive, MD
	Herbert Peterson, MD
2000	Mary D'Alton, MD
	Karen B. Nelson, MD
	Thomas G. Stovall, MD, MBA
2001	John A. Collins, MD
	Patrick Duff, MD
	Washington Hill, MD
	Baha Sibai, MD
	Bruce Zwiebel, MD
	Charles E. Cox, MD
	Julie Larkin, MD
2002	Murray A. Freedman, MD
	William D. Schlaff, MD
	Jeffrey P. Phelan, MD, MBA
	Ruben A. Quintero, MD
2003	Mark I. Evans, MD
	Thomas G. Stovall, MD, MBA

2004   Paul A. Gluck, MD
            Kenneth R. Kellner, MD, PhD
            Theodore Rosen, MD
            Jacques Rioux, MD
            C. Robert Stanhope, MD

2005   Willy Davila, MD
            Kenneth R. Kellner, MD, PhD
            Steve D. McCarus, MD
            Glenn A. Miller, PhD
            Robert R. Ruffolo Jr., PhD
            Lee P. Schulman, MD

2006   Arnold W. Cohen, MD
            L. Michael Fleischman, CHC
            Fred M. Howard, MD
            Daniel R. Mishell, MD
            Baha Sibai, MD
            Celso Silva, MD

2007   John O. Delancey, MD
            Steven D. McCarus, MD
            Charles N. Paidas, MD
            Michael J. Paidas, MD
            Lee P. Schulman, MD

2008   Pedro Escobar, MD
            Larry Glazerman, MD, MBA
            Paul A. Gluck, MD
            Daniel R. Mishell, MD
            Raul Ordorica, MD

2009   Ronald T. Burkman, MD
            Fred Turek, PhD
            Patricia J. Bickle

2010   Fredric Frigoletto, MD
            Paul A. Gluck, MD
            Mark R. Hughes, MD, PhD
            James W. Orr, MD
            Maureen Whelihan, MD

Introduction to Chapter 4

The Classic Department
Expansion and Growth

Prior to the late 1980s, medical insurance was one of two types: (1) the indemnity variety in which the patient paid the doctor's total bill and it was their responsibility to collect their money from the insurance company and (2), principally, the Blue Cross and Blue Shield (by far the largest private nonprofit insurance carrier) in whose participating program the physician was paid directly by the insurance company, although at a lower rate. In most instances, 80 percent of physician charges were paid by the insurance carrier and 20 percent by the patient.

Shortly after the 1992 presidential election, the Clinton administration attempted to reform health care along the universal-coverage model. Their failure to do so resulted in the concept of managed competition, with formation of HMOs, PPOs, and point of service organizations (POS) on either a discounted fee for service or capitated basis. Control of care and the amount of medical reimbursement for patients in this model was transferred to the insurance company rather than the physician. An emphasis on reducing costs became the watchword, and many insurance carriers put as one impediment in the way of getting medical care the gatekeeper concept. Gatekeepers were generally primary-care physicians, and they controlled access to specialists.

This was a particular problem for obstetricians and gynecologists. Older women often had a primary-care physician in the form of a family practitioner or internist. Younger women by contrast, who are usually healthy, saw their OB-GYN doctors for their yearly gynecologic exam and their care during pregnancy. Access to an OB-GYN doctor now had to be on a referral basis from primary-care physicians, for whom most of these healthy young women rarely had need.

Fearful of losing numbers and control of patients, as well as federal funding now emphasizing the concept of primary care, the American Congress of Obstetricians and Gynecologists now lobbied to have obstetrician-gynecologists recognized as primary-care doctors rather than specialists. Residency training in obstetrics and gynecology was altered in academic centers (with which by this time essentially all residency programs were affiliated) by shortening or eliminating resident exposure to the subspecialties of reproductive endocrinology and infertility, gynecologic oncology, and maternal-fetal medicine. They allocated that time to primary-care endeavors in family medicine and internal medicine services. While this anomaly lasted only ten years or so, by the mid-1990s, obstetrician-gynecologists thought of themselves as specialists as well as primary-care physicians.

These were challenges that the new chairman, Dr. William Spellacy, faced while endeavoring to expand the breadth and depth of services offered by the department.

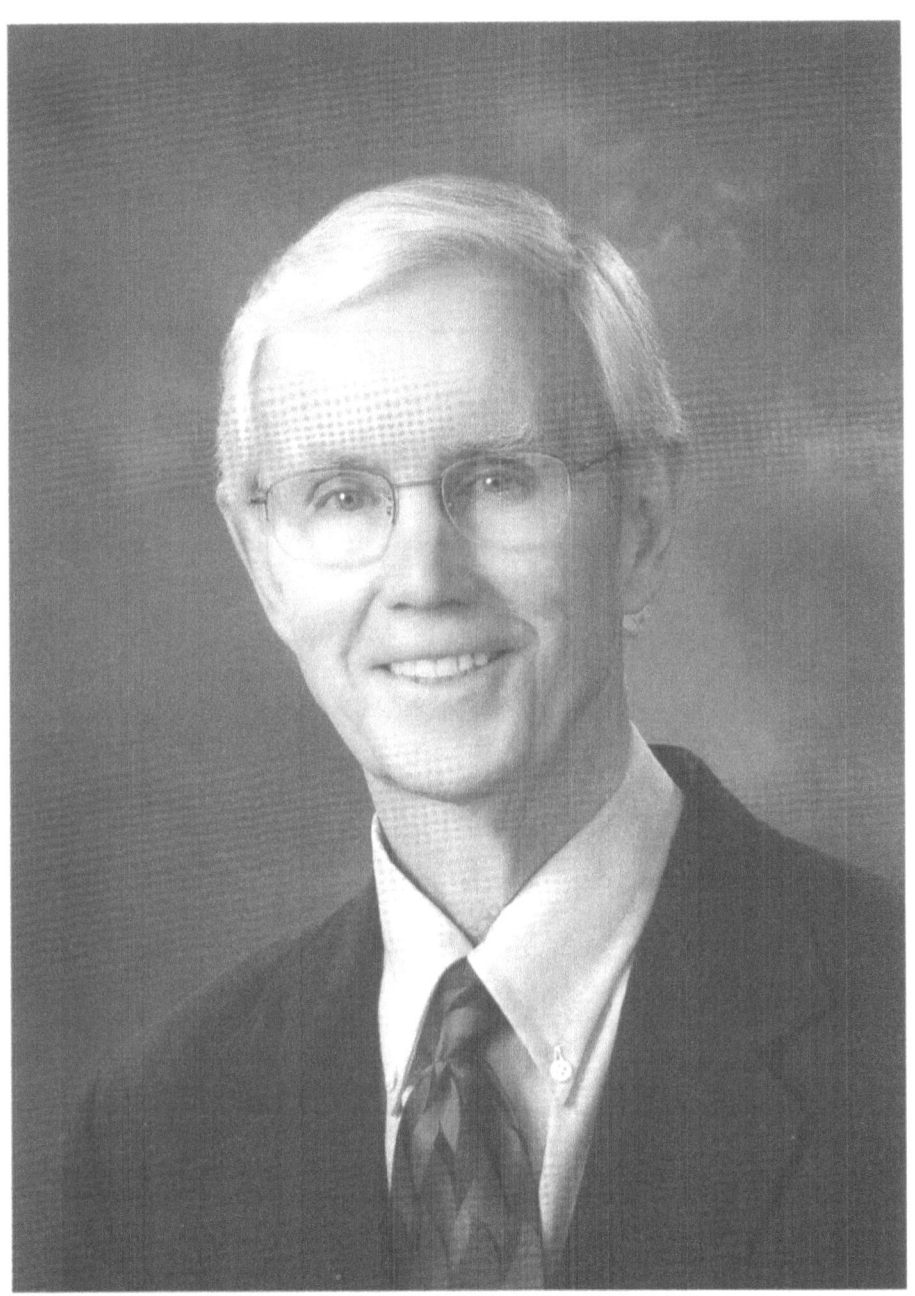

William N. Spellacy, MD

CHAPTER 4

William N. Spellacy, MD

by Michael Parsons, MD, MBA

William Nelson Spellacy was born May 10, 1934, in Saint Paul, Minnesota. He attended the University of Minnesota for his undergraduate education. Dr. Spellacy continued at the University of Minnesota for his medical education, achieving Alpha Omega Alpha status for academic excellence and successfully completing his residency in obstetrics and gynecology at the University of Minnesota under chairmen Nicholson J. Eastman, MD, and John L. McKelvey, MD.

His professional academic career began as a faculty member of the University of Minnesota and then at the University of Miami, rapidly advancing to the academic rank of professor. Despite his not being chairman of the department, many residents at the time considered themselves "Spellacy's Boys." As a result of his excellence in teaching, innovative research activities with significant contributions to the peer-reviewed literature, and recognized clinical expertise, Dr. Spellacy was appointed chairman at the Department of Obstetrics and Gynecology at the University of Florida while still in his 30s—a remarkable feat in its day.

During this time, as Dr. Spellacy was gaining greater prominence on a national and international level, he was recruited to play a larger role in the direction of the future of obstetrics and gynecology. He was one of the main architects of the design and formation of the three new subspecialties in obstetrics and gynecology: maternal-fetal medicine, reproductive endocrinology and infertility, and gynecologic oncology. These provided physicians an opportunity to acquire additional training, thus advancing patient care and research activity in these subspecialty fields. Dr. Spellacy chose to become certified in maternal medicine but maintained interest in all areas.

During most of the 1970s, Dr. Spellacy continued as the chairman of obstetrics and gynecology at the University of Florida. At that time, the three obstetrics fetal gynecology university chairmen in Florida (William A. Little, University of Miami; James M. Ingram Jr., University of South Florida [USF]; and Dr. Spellacy, University of Florida) met periodically to discuss problems, curriculum, state funding, and other issues. They would meet in a central place, which was Tampa. Dr. Ingram would have them meet at Tampa General Hospital or sometimes at his beach house, Journey's End, in Boca Grande on Gasparilla Island. Because of these many visits, Dr. Spellacy knew Tampa well, both the city and the Obstetrics and Gynecology Department.

In 1979, Dr. Spellacy moved to Chicago to head the Department of Obstetrics and Gynecology at the University of Illinois. Under his leadership, the department achieved national prominence in research, education, and patient care. During this time, his professional career continued to blossom. He was elected president of some of the most important national organizations in obstetrics and gynecology, including the Society of Perinatal Obstetricians, Association of Professors of Gynecology and Obstetrics, and Society for Gynecologic Investigation. Additionally, he continued as both a board examiner of resident graduates and also as director for the American Board of Obstetrics and Gynecology.

When Dr. Ingram decided to step down from his department chairmanship in 1987, the chairman of the search committee, Dr. Lou Barness, who was also the chairman of the Department of Pediatrics at USF Morsani College of Medicine, contacted Dr. Spellacy to see if he would visit and consider being a candidate for the obstetrics and gynecology chair. At that time, he was enjoying his position at the University of Illinois and had no plans to leave Chicago, but he also had enough sand in his shoes from time in Florida to look at this new opportunity. Therefore, he accepted the invitation to visit on July 1, 1987, and was shown around by Dr. Ronald Kaufman, who was vice president for health at USF. Dr. Spellacy provided a list of things he felt the department needed. Dr. Kaufman and the CEO at Tampa General Hospital, Newell France, responded by producing almost everything on that list in terms of space, equipment, and money, and he accepted the offer to become the second chairman of the Department of Obstetrics and Gynecology of USF Morsani College of Medicine in March of 1988 and moved to Tampa. His first day at work was July 1, 1988.

Moving to Tampa to practice and teach was exciting, and he looked forward to seeing former residents now in practice there, including Dr. Beth Benson (University of Illinois resident) and Dr. Tony Messina and Dr. Nicholas Fallieras (University of Florida residents). When he arrived in Tampa in July, the faculty was separated geographically in several buildings, including the One Davis Patient Office Building, the USF campus, Tampa General Hospital, and the Moffitt Cancer Center. In general, each division was together at one site, but the department was fragmented into several locations, and they infrequently met. The Maternal-Fetal Medicine Division was headed by Dr. Robert Knupple with members Drs. William O'Brien, Kathy Porter, and Jeff Angel. The Oncology Division was headed by Dr. Denis Cavanagh and included Drs. Bill Roberts, Mitchel Hoffman, and Jim LaPolla. The Reproductive Endocrine Division was headed by Dr. George Maroulis. The Gynecology Division was headed by James M. Ingram Jr. and included Drs. J. K. Williams and Pete Bouis.

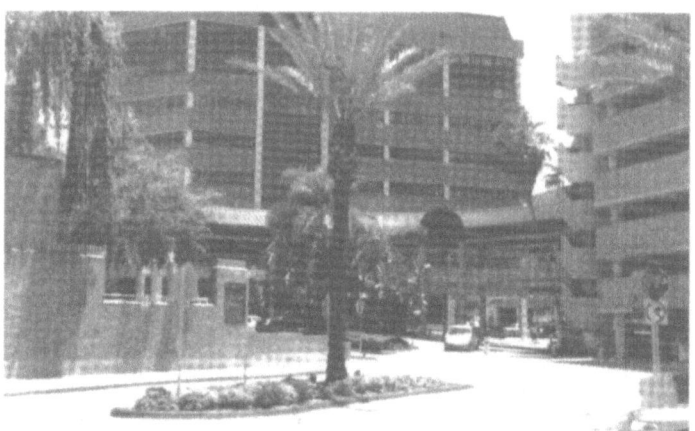

Harbourside Medical Towers, circa 1999

One of his first priorities was to bring these faculty members to one site and establish unity and a "department mentality." He leased the entire undeveloped fifth floor of the Harbourside Medical Tower (HMT) next to Tampa General Hospital (TGH) and with an architect, drew up plans for its development of twelve thousand square feet of academic space. The department already had a private outpatient space on the fourth floor of HMT, and it was very convenient for the faculty to move from their academic office to go see patients. In the new academic space, individual faculty offices were on the outside of the floor, so windows were available. There was storage, work space, and a mail room on the inside areas of the floor. At one end, there was built a large library-teaching room with an adjoining kitchen area for staff to have lunch and to service the conference room for some of its lunches. Bookshelves were built in the library and in the faculty offices, enhancing an academic atmosphere. He then had a search done to purchase bound OB-GYN journals back to volume 1 of each to stock the library and compiled a complete set of journals, including *Obstetrics & Gynecology*, *American Journal of Obstetrics & Gynecology*, *Obstetrical & Gynecological Survey*, *Fertility and Sterility*, *Contraception*, *Journal of Reproductive Medicine*, and *Journal of the Society for Gynecologic Investigation*, as well as many textbooks in all areas of obstetrics and gynecology. This was a great asset for the department, and it was used by medical students, residents, fellows, and faculty for study, research, and teaching. The room was equipped with audiovisual systems, podium, tables, and chairs. The room was dedicated as the James M. Ingram Library, and Dr. Ingram's portrait was hung there.

Dr. Spellacy's next project was to expand the department's basic laboratory-research space. There were wet laboratories totaling of 1,400 square feet at the USF campus assigned to the department, but that was felt to be too small. Dr. Kaufman and Mr. Newell France, the hospital administrator, freed up adequate space in TGH's first floor, which was formerly the pathology-laboratory space. This space was renovated and equipped with benches, hoods, and removable equipment, like centrifuges, freezers, gamma counters, and spectrophotometers. It added an additional 3,200 square feet of research space to the department, which was ready for use in 1989.

Another problem to resolve was the lack of ambulatory clinic space for the department. There was an approved four-year residency program with five positions per year and twenty residents. In addition, twelve to sixteen third-year medical students were around at all times on their clerkship. There was minimal outpatient care being done in one small 3,500-square-foot first-floor clinic in the back of TGH. In a search to find other potential clinic space, Dr. Spellacy became aware that TGH at one time had been physically several facilities: a large hospital on Davis Island and several smaller buildings including a hospital on North Thirtieth Street. The Thirtieth Street hospital had eventually been closed and sat vacant for many years. With the help of the TGH administration and key individuals, including Dee Jeffers and Margaret Swanson, a visit to Tallahassee with legislators to explain the need for money to renovate a part of the old TGH Thirtieth Street hospital into a modern women-and-infants outpatient-care facility resulted in about one million dollars of aid. The new unit was named Genesis and provided an additional 24,000 square feet of space for women's ambulatory, comprehensive health care, including ultrasound imaging, colposcopy, continuity clinics for residents in obstetrics and gynecology, family-planning clinics, pediatric-newborn clinics, and much more.

In its early years, the clinic was directed by Dr. Ronald Chez, who joined the faculty, having previously been chairman of OB-GYN at Penn State College of Medicine at Hershey and had developed an interest in ambulatory care. Genesis remains as an active TGH outpatient facility for the department and has more than thirty-five thousand visits per year to provide primary and tertiary health care in one location to low-income women and children.

After stepping down as chairman, James M. Ingram, MD, remained in the department, continuing his excellence in patient care and mentoring the junior faculty. He died on November 7, 1989, just over a year after resigning as chairman. With the generous help of his many friends, former students, residents, and patients, Dr. Spellacy spearheaded an effort to endow a million-dollar chair in the department in Dr. Ingram's name. This is now and always will be held by the chairperson of the department.

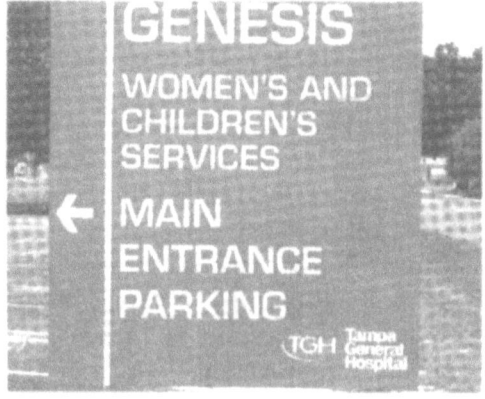

Sign for Genesis Clinic

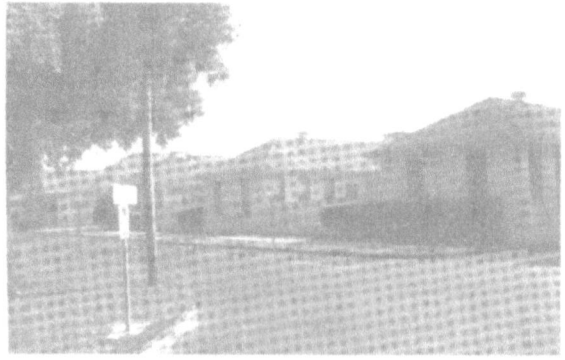

Genesis Clinic, outside view

In 1997, it became apparent to Dr. Spellacy that many women who were being seen at Tampa General Hospital and in the Genesis clinic were inmates from the Hillsborough County Jail. Their care was fragmented because of their incarceration, yet it was the department's desire and responsibility to achieve good medical outcomes for their pregnancies and gynecologic problems. Dr. Spellacy met with Joann Carver, RN, a director of women's health at the jails, and developed a plan whereby all incarcerated pregnant women in the three jails would be moved and stay in one pod at the Hillsborough County Falkenberg Jail. Dr. Spellacy would visit every two weeks to provide prenatal, postpartum, and gynecologic care. All necessary hospitalization for delivery or gynecologic surgery would be done at Tampa General Hospital, thus providing continuity of care. That plan is still in place, and the women who are incarcerated in Hillsborough County now receive high-quality, comprehensive obstetrics and gynecologic care.

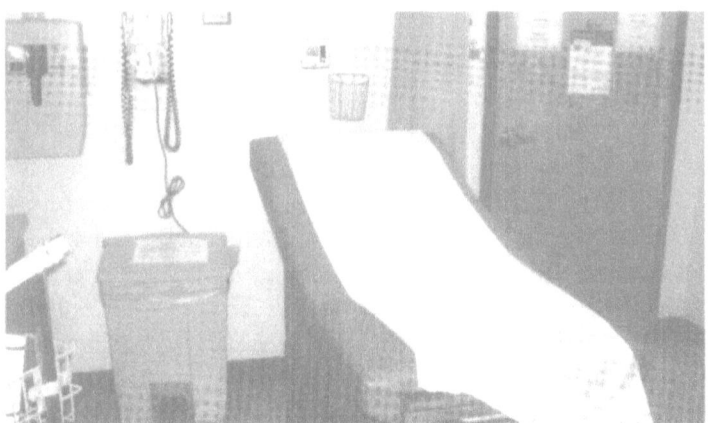

Genesis Clinic, inside view

In 1992, the Perinatal Outreach Program started and was directed by Dr. Spellacy. The program features a team of specialized perinatal physicians who travel to four clinics, including public-health units in Bartow, Dade City, New Port Richey, and Ruskin. The team—including a maternal-fetal-medicine physician, a perinatal nurse coordinator, a genetics counselor, and ultrasonographers—provides patients in these rural communities with access to specialized prenatal care for women with high-risk pregnancies.

"The three biggest problems in the health-care system are access, cost, and quality" is a statement and belief that Dr. Spellacy has expressed and worked to improve in many ways. He has spent much of his professional life making sure that women in the Tampa Bay and surrounding areas had access to the best medical care possible. As is evident from the above accomplishments, he has had considerable success in addressing these problems, greatly benefiting the community.

Another issue which Dr. Spellacy faced was the increasing number of women entering the program. While in earlier years, more women interested in medicine engaged a career in nursing, after the "consciousness revolution" of the late 1960s and 1970s of which woman's liberation was a part, increasing numbers of women began entering medical school. In the early days of the department, over 90 percent of medical students were men; by 2000, this percentage was about 50 percent (table 6). While in the early days of the department, about 90 percent of OB-GYN residents were men, by 2000, approximately 70 percent were women (table 7). The practicalities of this social shift were handled with his usual aplomb and common sense.

The USF faculty continued their academic activities over the years since 1988 by teaching medical students, residents, fellows, and practitioners in the community, the latter principally by the annual Midwinter Seminar and grand rounds. A major effort of the faculty during these years has been the teaching and training of the residents. Excellent, top-ranked medical students from all over the United States came into the OB-GYN residency program, and the graduating residents have gone into practice in many different states from California to New York and Illinois to Louisiana. An impressive fact is that all USF OB-GYN residents have passed the American Board of Obstetrics and Gynecology examinations and are certified in the specialty. The department faculty continued to be active not only in teaching and in providing patient care, but have also expanded their productivity in performing clinical and basic research.

Dr. Spellacy continued his prodigious output of important medical literature while at USF, with research activities that provided new information to advance all areas of health care and improve teaching to students and residents. His breadth of interest in pregnancy-related and women's health care ranged from diabetes mellitus in pregnancy, hormonal influences of pregnancy, contraception, intrauterine growth restriction, biochemical and biophysical fetal monitoring, management of labor, prevention of preterm-delivery complications, and multiple pregnancies and range from operative obstetrics to evaluating teaching effectiveness of medical students and residents, to list just a few examples. His contributions to the literature have been most impressive in both quality and quantity, with over five hundred peer-reviewed articles, eighty book chapters, and ten books resulting from his efforts. He has been well recognized for his expertise and is sought as a lecturer on the national and international stage for his clear, comprehensive, and common-sense approach to conveying information and knowledge.

During his time as chairman at USF, Dr. Spellacy was the recipient of numerous honors and recognitions, including being elected to the Institute of Medicine, the health arm of the National Academy of Sciences, one of the highest honors in medicine. This prestigious organization elects only the most distinguished individuals in the fields of health and medicine.

Dr. Spellacy is one of the rare individuals in academic medicine who have excelled in all areas of the field: patient care, education, and advancing knowledge through research and new discoveries. Always aware of having the patient as the central focus, he has influenced and served as a role model for generations of students, residents, faculty, and colleagues as a physician who strives and succeeds to make long-lasting improvements in health care.

Having relinquished the chairmanship in 2002, Dr. Spellacy continues with his full-time clinical and teaching responsibilities as professor and director of the residency program and provides valuable guidance and benefit of his experience to those who followed him.

The number of graduating residents, fellows, and those becoming faculty under Dr. Spellacy are seen in table 8. The faculty during Dr. Spellacy's tenure is displayed in table 9. The number of patients cared for and published research papers, chapters, and abstracts over the years of his chairmanship are seen in table 10.

Table 6

Percent of Women as First-Year Medical Students Over Time

Applicants Academic Year	Applicants Total	Matriculants Women as % of Total	Graduates Women as % of Total
1965–66	18,703	9.3%	6.9%
1970–71	24,987	11.1%	9.2%
1975–76	42,282	23.6%	16.2%
1980–81	36,083	28.7%	24.9%
1985–86	32,885	33.9%	30.8%
1990–91	29,241	38.5%	36.0%
1991–92	33,297	39.7%	36.1%
1992–93	37,402	41.6%	38.1%
1993–94	42,806	42.0%	38.0%
1994–95	45,360	41.9%	39.2%
1995–96	46,586	42.7%	40.9%
1996–97	46,965	42.7%	41.5%
1997–98	43,016	43.3%	41.7%
1998–99	40,996	44.3%	42.4%
1999–00	38,443	45.7%	42.5%
2000–01	37,088	45.8%	43.2%
2001–02	34,860	47.6%	44.2%
2002–03	33,625	49.2%	45.3%
2003–04	34,791	49.6%	45.9%
2004–05	35,735	49.5%	47.0%
2005–06	37,373	48.5%	48.7%
2006–07	39,108	48.6%	49.1%
2007–08	42,315	48.3%	49.3%
2008–09	42,231	47.8%	48.8%

Source: AAMC 2011

Table 7

Percent of OB-GYN Residents Who Are Female

Year	Total # of Programs (NRMP)	Total OB-GYN Residents	Females	% Female	% Positions Matched (NRMP)
2010	237				99.6
2009	245				99.5
2008	247	4,815	3,755	78.0	99.0
2007	249	4,770	3,657	76.7	99.5
2006	250	4,739	3,596	75.9	97.9
2005	252	4,720	3,568	75.6	94.7
2004	252	4,703	3,504	74.5	93.3
2003	256	4,681	3,483	74.4	91.2
2002	254	4,656	3,433	73.7	93.8
2001	254	4,701	3,357	71.4	92.4
2000	254	4,679	3,255	69.6	92.1
1999	256	4,710	3,165	67.2	93.1
1998	262	4,810	3,098	64.4	95.6
1997	264	4,881	3,055	62.6	97.1
1996	267	4,941	2,972	60.1	96.9
1995		5,007	2,899	57.9	96.5
1994		5,046	2,828	56.0	98.7
1993		5,074	2,689	53.0	98.3
1992		4,843	2,415	50.7	96.6
1991		4,526	2,316	48.3	97.2
1990		4,764	2,216	46.5	97.0
1989		4,655	2,172	46.7	94.9
1988		4,426	2,172	47.2	94.1
1987		4,520	2,133	46.5	89.9
1986		4,525	2,066	43.4	92.9
1985		4,658	1,942	41.8	94.9
1984		4,704	1,824	38.9	97.0
1983		4,631	1,758	36.5	95.0
1982		4,702	1,694	34.4	93.0
1981		4,705	1,583	32.9	91.0
1980		4,221	1,408	30.6	88.0
1979		4,517	1,260	27.9	

1978		4,258	1,013	23.8	
1977		4,141	789	19.3	
1976		3,896	623	16.0	
1975		3,772	549	14.6	

Sources:

JAMA medical education issues, ACOG manpower data, NRMP data, 2009 number of programs from NRMP.

Table 8

Residents Serving Under William N. Spellacy, MD

Year	Resident	Medical School	
1989	Michael W. Jaeger, MD	U. of South Florida	
	Mary Lee Josey, MD	U. of South Florida	
	Matthew R. Mervis, MD	U. of Michigan	
	Shirley K. Sawai, MD	U. of South Florida	M
	Stephen G. Smith, MD	U. of Florida	
1990	Evan M. Collins, MD	U. of Tennessee	
	Michael A. Finan, MD	Louisiana State U.	O/F
	Steven L. Greenberg, MD	U. of Texas	
	Linda McClain, MD	E. Carolina U.	
	Sheri A. Owens, MD	U. of S. Alabama	F
1991	Jorge J. Lense, MD	U. of South Florida	
	Micheal G. Mastry, MD	U. of Pittsburgh	
	Timothy D. O'Leary, MD	U. of Missouri	M
	Kathleen A. Reilly, MD	U. of South Florida	
	Andrew C. Villa Jr., MD	U. of South Florida	
1992	Nicolas M. Colorado, MD	U. of South Florida	
	Jodi L. Holbrook, MD	U. of Iowa	
	Craig S. Kalter, MD	U. of South Florida	M
	James C. Mayer, MD	Tulane University	R/F
	Stratton N. Sterghos Jr., MD	U. of South Florida	

1993	Elbridge F. Bills, MD	Emory School of Medicine	
	Gregory W. Chen, MD	U. of Illinois	
	Steven L. DeCesare, MD	New Jersey Medical School	O/F
	Micah S. Harris, MD	U. of South Florida	
	Donna M. Pinelli, MD	Medical College of Virginia	O
	Jack J. Wilson, MD	U. of Alabama	
1994	Hector Arango, MD	U. of South Florida	O
	Madelyn Butler, MD	U. of Florida	
	Scott C. Dresdan, MD	U. of South Florida	
	D. Ashley Hill, MD	U. of South Florida	
	Catherine Lynch, MD	U. of South Florida	F
	Janet Vodra, MD	U. of Miami	
1995	Robert M. Dacus, MD	U. of North Carolina	
	Valerie M. Goldfain, MD	U. of Illinois	
	Sylvia T. Goodwin, MD	U. of Miami	
	Duncan F. Guedon, MD	U. of Mississippi	
	Christine M. Kneer, MD	U. of South Florida	F
	Armando L. Rojas, MD	Mercer University	
1996	Michael L. Cacciatore, MD	U. of South Florida	
	Janie E. Furer, MD	U. of Illinois	
	Alecia E. Graves, MD	U. of Louisville	
	Allahyar Jazayeri, MD, PhD	U. of Texas Medical Branch	M
	Raymond A. Mathews, MD	Wake Forest University	
	Greg A. Towsley, MD	U. of South Florida	
1997	N. Donald Diebel, MD	U. of South Florida	
	Julia A. Heffron, MD	Medical College of Georgia	
	Eric B. Jacoby, MD	Tulane University	
	Jean McClintock, MD	Texas A&M University	
	Todd D. Meisinger, MD	Saint Louis University	
	Sandra Murphy, MD	U. of South Florida	
1998	John F. Bagnasco, MD	U. of South Carolina	
	Richard J. Cardosi, MD	U. of Tennessee	O
	Heidi E. Hagler-Arnold, MD	U. of Tennessee	
	Kimberly A. Huffman, MD	U. of Florida	

	Suzanne T. Mann-Icely, MD	U. of Florida	
	Cherrie A. Rulka-Morris, MD	New Jersey Medical School	
1999	Murray F. Dweck, MD	Tulane University	
	Molly M. Long, MD	U. of Illinois	
	Melissa M. Moore, MD	U. of Iowa	
	Scott E. Musinski, MD	U. of Connecticut	
	Laura B. Politz, MD	Louisiana State University	
	Renee B. Schwandt, MD	U. of South Florida	
2000	Renda K. Knapp, MD	U. of South Florida	
	Jennifer D. Campbell, MD	U. Texas, San Antonio	
	Jennifer R. Gilby, MD	U. Florida	
	Diana C. Hicks, MD	Eastern Virginia Medical School	
	Catherine L. Johnson, MD	Brody School of Medicine	
	Robert F. Lemert, MD	U. South Carolina	
2001	Ingrid W. Brown, MD	U. of Texas Medical Branch	
	Rosemary P. Cardosi, MD	U. of South Florida	
	Sheila S. Devanesan, MD	U. of South Florida	
	Ronnie L. Frankel, MD	U. of South Florida	
	Joan M. McCarthy, MD	UMDNJ–Robert Wood Johnson Medical School	
	Nancy S. Miller, MD	U. of South Florida	
	Wendy M. Riggs, MD	U. of S. Alabama	
2002	Kevin H. Brown, MD	Med Col. of Georgia	
	Carol G. Cox, MD	U. of Maryland	F
	Carrie A. Grounds, MD	U. of Missouri	
	Leesa A. Kaufman, MD	U. of South Florida	
	R. Scott Lucidi, MD	Saint Louis University	R
	Nancy A. MacLaurin, MD	U. of Connecticut	
2003	Amy W. Dietelhorst, MD	Saint Louis University	
	Jonathan H. Griner, MD	U. of Maryland	
	Kiera M. Irvin, MD	U. of South Florida	
	Keisha L. Loftin, MD	U. of Texas, San Antonio	
	Parmelee Thatcher, MD	U. of South Florida	

	Jennifer B. Thrasher, MD	U. Miami	
2004	Maria Baker, MD	U. of South Florida	
	Odette C. Daley, MD	Morehouse School of Medicine	
	Sylvia S. Siegfried, MD	U. of Florida	
	Stephen J. Tebes, MD	U. of Florida	
	Emanuel C. Trabuco, MD	U. of Colorado	R

Fellowships

M—Maternal-Fetal Medicine
O—Oncology
R—Reproductive Endocrinology and Infertility
U—Urogynecology
F—Faculty

Table 9

Faculty Serving Under William N. Spellacy, MD*

Faculty Member

Alice Rhoton-Vlasak, MD
Angela Keating, MD
Anna Parsons, MD
Carol Cox, MD
Denis Cavanagh, MD
Catherine Lynch, MD
Edward Grendys, MD
Irvin Strathman, MD
J. K. Williams, MD
James Fiorica, MD
James Mayer, MD
Jeanne Becker, PhD
Jeryl Natofsky, MD
Joan McCarthy, MD
John Tsibris, PhD
Johnathan Lancaster, MD
Judith Krammer, MD
Karen Bruder, MD
Lauri Hochberg, MD
Lorraine Bevilaqua, MD
Lynn Boardman, MD
Marcelo Barrionueva, MD
Mark Mclean, PhD
Mark Williams, MD
Michael Parsons, MD
Pierre Bouis, MD
Robert Wenham, MD
Ronald Chez, MD
Sean Tedjarati, MD
Shelly Holmstrom, MD
Stanley Gould, MD
Timothy Yeko, MD
William O'Brien, MD
William Roberts, MD
William Spellacy, MD

---

*   *In order by first name*

Table 10

Departmental Activity in 1990 through 2008

Obstetrics Clinical Care Gynecologic Clinical Care Academic Productivity

Year	# FTE Faculty	Total Deliveries	Cesarean Sections	%	Major OR	Minor OR	Total OR	Paper Chapters	Abstracts
1990	22	6,895	1,062	15.4	1,076	971	2,047	62	36
1991	24	7,075	1,013	14.3	1,131	419	1,550	62	45
1992	24	5,386	826	15.3	1,054	458	1,512	48	34
1993	25	3,953	644	16.3	1,061	527	1,598	51	36
1994	24	2,969	498	16.8	1,133	498	1,631	55	42
1995	24	2,656	481	18.1	1,153	552	1,705	69	40
1996	27	3,245	668	20.6	1,125	493	1,618	57	24
1997	26	3,174	673	21.2	1,120	651	1,771	56	45
1998	27	3,158	619	19.6	1,019	496	1,515	57	23
1999	24	3,254	699	21.5	1,031	521	1,552	64	23
2000	22	3,509	735	20.1	1,037	450	1,487	49	21
2001	23	3,810	967	25.4	1,234	477	1,711	38	10
2002	23	4,383	1,018	23.2	1,078	414	1,492	32	10
2003	21	4,232	1,045	25.0	1,303	385	1,688	26	12
2004	20	4,523	1,226	27.1	1,398	555	1,953	33	8
2005	31	4,831	1,324	27.4	1,454	564	2,018	27	14
2006	31	5,391	1,587	29.4	1,599	706	2,305	19	14
2007	35	5,457	1,697	31.1	1,490	733	2,223	32	19
2008	33	5,664	1,765	31.2	1,695	674	2,369	22	10

CHAPTER 5

Accelerated Growth

USF Gynecologic Oncology
An Abbreviated History

by *Mitchel Hoffman, MD*

The modern era of gynecologic oncology dates back approximately one hundred years to the development of a radical operation for the treatment of cervical cancer and the subsequent use of radiation therapy for the management of this same disease. Pelvic exenteration for cervical cancer and radical debulking operations for ovarian cancer were described in the 1950s. Chemotherapy agents were being developed at that time, which were found to cure trophoblastic disease and improve survival in ovarian-cancer patients, especially when a cytoreductive operation removing most or all visible tumor had been performed. During that time, gynecologic cancer surgery at major medical centers was performed by gynecologists and/or general surgeons with a special interest in these disease processes.

In May 1968, like-minded fellows of the American Congress of Obstetricians and Gynecologists met to discuss the potential to form a society consisting of obstetrician-gynecologists whose major interest was gynecologic cancer. In January 1969, interested parties were gathered to formalize the creation of the Society of Gynecologic Oncology. In January 1970, the first Annual Meeting of the Society of Gynecologic Oncology was convened. In 1972, the subspecialties of gynecologic oncology, reproductive endocrinology, and maternal-fetal medicine were formally approved by

---

the American Board of Medical Specialties. The first written and oral examinations for certification for special competence in gynecologic oncology were given in 1974 at which time, Dr. Cavanagh was certified.

In 1978, Dr. Denis Cavanagh, one of the original fifty-seven founding members of the Society of Gynecologic Oncology, was recruited by Dr. James M. Ingram Jr. to create a Division of Gynecologic Oncology at USF.

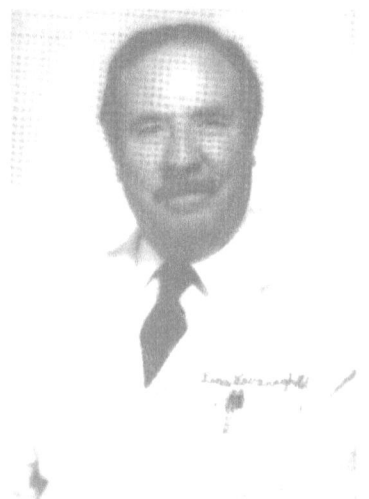

Dr. Denis Cavanagh

Dr. Cavanagh came to Tampa with his first fellow, Dr. Hora Praphat, and his longtime research associate, Dr. Papaneni Rao. The following year, his second fellow—Dr. John Shepherd—was recruited from London. The division's practice, research, and education programs thrived and created a vastly improved new standard of care for women suffering from gynecologic cancer in Southwest Florida. Through ironfisted leadership, an unwavering commitment to medical practice, research and education, and a legendary sense of humor, Denis Cavanagh directed the USF Division of Gynecologic Oncology for twenty years. He created a national and international reputation for gynecologic cancer care at USF. Dr. Cavanagh's greatest legacy is the education and commitment to medicine he instilled in the fellows, residents, and medical students who were fortunate enough to train under him.

Many other faculty members were instrumental in developing and promulgating the USF Division of Gynecologic Oncology. Many years of outstanding research came out of Papaneni Rao's lab and then, later, the labs of Jeannie Becker, Santo Nicosia, and Johnathan Lancaster. Hora Praphat, an exceptionally capable clinician, helped Dr. Cavanagh get the clinical program started, subsequently entering private practice in Tampa. William Roberts was recruited, having completed his fellowship in California, to join the division in 1982. Fellows and residents who have trained under Dr. Roberts hold him in the highest esteem as a superior gynecologic-oncology clinician and educator.

Denis Cavanagh was a charming Scotsman with an unusual sense of humor, who did his medical training at the University of Glasgow in Scotland. In 1958, he came to the United States, completing a fellowship in gynecologic oncology at MD Anderson Cancer Center in Houston and then joined the faculty of the University of Miami Miller School of Medicine, where he remained rising to the rank of professor. He had many clinical interests, ranging from hypertension in pregnancy to gynecologic malignancies, which were his special interest. He left the University of Miami to become chairman of the Department of Obstetrics and Gynecology at Saint Louis University– School of Medicine and, subsequently, chairman of the Department of Obstetrics and Gynecology of the school of medicine at the University of Tasmania, an island just south of Australia. He returned to Saint Louis as chairman and spearheaded the building of a women's center for the university as he had done in Tasmania and was recruited by James Ingram to initiate the vision of gynecologic oncology at USF.

Dr. Cavanagh was an outstanding individual who was an organizing, normal, or honorary member of many national and international societies. He authored or coauthored four textbooks, forty textbook chapters, and over 225 peer-reviewed articles in medical journals. He was a skilled surgeon and an ebullient leader. Dr. Cavanagh became disabled in 1999 and retired in Sarasota.

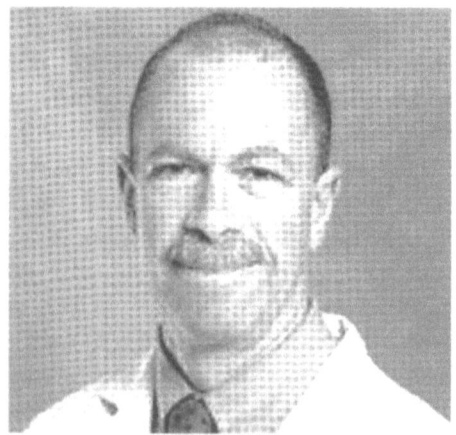

Dr. Mitchel Hoffman

Dr. Mitchel Hoffman, one of Dr. Cavanagh's most outstanding fellows and an exquisite surgeon, was named division head and fellowship director and continues to serve in that capacity to this day. Dr. Hoffman completed his residency and *gynecologic* fellowship in the Department of Obstetrics and Gynecology at the University of South Florida. He has authored over two hundred refereed publications and book chapters, is an examiner for the basic OB-GYN and gynecologic-oncology boards, and is the Teasley-Tampa general professor in USF gynecologic oncology.

In 1980, a state-funded cancer institute was opened in Tampa under the auspices of the legislature and named after the then-speaker of the house, H. Lee Moffitt, a Tampa native and one of youngest house leaders in Florida history. The Moffitt Cancer Center grew over time to become one of the nation's foremost cancer institutes and has been designated as such by the National Cancer Institute.

Dr. James Fiorica joined the USF Division of Gynecologic Oncology in 1989 and became program leader of gynecologic oncology at the Moffitt Cancer Center in 1996. Jim developed an outstanding program at the H. Lee Moffitt Cancer Center as well as a large GOG consortium.

Moffitt was a USF-affiliated hospital at that time, and the gynecologic-oncology program at Moffitt existed in concert with the *gyn*-oncology services at Tampa General Gynecologic Hospital in serving as the basis of the USF *gyn*-oncology program and fellowship and gynecologic resident teaching exposure.

A state institution chartered separately from USF, it naturally followed that the interests of Moffitt sometimes did not coincide with USF, and the relationship over the years varied in its cordially, depth, and reach of faculty involvement.

Sensing an increasing chasm between USF and Moffitt, Drs. Hoffman and Fiorica worked hard to forge a relationship that would allow the fellowship to survive politically and practically induced separation of the two facilities. In 2004, the Moffitt Cancer Center became an independent institution. In 2005, Jim Fiorica went into private practice in Sarasota. Before leaving, Jim had the Moffitt gynecologic-oncology program firmly situated. Johnathan Lancaster, MD, PhD, trained at Duke University, is its present program leader.

Currently, USF and Moffitt function as two independent gynecologic-oncology services—two sites supporting a single fellowship program. The fellowship training program, one of forty-three in the nation, maintains the tradition of excellence that began in 1978. Jointly, USF and Moffitt continue to lead the region with a nationally recognized program for the care of women afflicted with gynecologic cancer. Clinical trials and basic science-research programs (especially, externally funded ovarian-cancer research in the labs of Santo Nicosia and Johnathan Lancaster) are cutting-edge. The patient care, education, and research carried out by the division are a great tribute to Dr. Cavanagh and USF and bode well for an extremely bright future.

Other outstanding individuals who have worked in and contributed to the advancement of the USF Division of Gynecologic Oncology include John Kavanagh, James LaPolla, Tom McDonald, Phillip Townsend, Ed Grendys, and Robyn Sayer.

At the time of this writing, the USF Division of Gynecologic Oncology will be graduating its twenty-sixth fellow in an outstanding group of gynecologic oncologists of which the OB-GYN Department is truly proud. As a group, they comprise the Denis Cavanagh Society. The division also takes pride in the role it has played in the education of the USF obstetrics-and-gynecology residents. For the future, the USF Division of Gynecologic Oncology will continue to uphold the tradition of excellence in patient care, education, and research that was begun by Dr. Cavanagh.

The Division of Maternal-Fetal Medicine

by J. K. Williams, MD

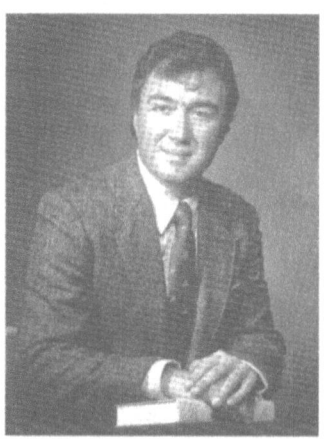

Dr. Robert Knuppel

The American Board of Obstetrics and Gynecology (ABOG) was founded in 1927, six years before the official formation of the American Board of Medical Specialties (ABMS). By 1972, ABOG formed the first subspecialties in OB-GYN, and within a few short years, Dr. Ingram created the USF Division of Maternal-Fetal Medicine and recruited Robert Knupple, MD, MPH, from Tufts University, to head the division. Born and raised in New Jersey, Dr. Knupple was educated at Georgetown University and the New Jersey Medical School. His residency and fellowship were at Tufts University in Boston. Immediately following his fellowship, Dr. Knupple received his MPH from the Harvard School of Public Health and joined the USF faculty in 1979. He brought with him Jose Scerbo, MD—who had also been with him at Tufts—as his first faculty member. The division was committed to the board's original charge of advancing knowledge of the obstetrical, medical, and surgical complications of pregnancy and their effect on both the mother and the fetus by specialists who possess expertise in the most current diagnostic and treatment modalities used in the care of patients with complicated pregnancies.

From its inception in 1979 through 2003, the Maternal-Fetal Medicine Division was responsible for all obstetrical services in the department, encompassing research, education, and patient care. In fact, it was known as the Division of Maternal-Fetal Medicine and Obstetrics, caring for all pregnant women regardless of risk. It wasn't until 2003 that more routine obstetrics was handed over to the Division of General Obstetrics and Gynecology.

In the early years under the leadership of Dr. Knupple, the division's primary interest was bringing to USF research and education in the areas of prenatal diagnoses, obstetrical ultrasonography, and antenatal fetal testing. In 1982, Dr. Knupple, along with his research nurse, Joan Drukker, published the first textbook to come from the USF OB-GYN Department, *High Risk Obstetrics: A Team Approach*. Out of this collaboration came the perinatal grief-counseling program.

One of the first approved MFM fellowships in the United States was started at USF in 1980 with Dinesh Shah, MD, as its founding fellow. To get the fellowship off and running, the first four selected fellows, Drs. Shah, Pawan Rattan, Raul Montenegro, and J. K. Williams, were all experienced clinicians and functioned as faculty-fellows.

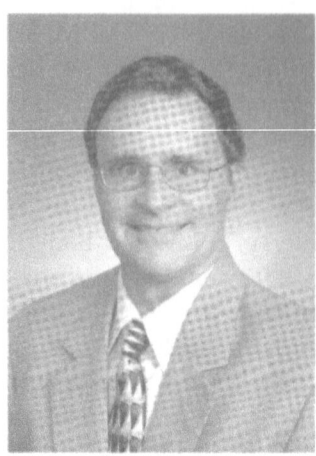

Dr. William O'Brien

As William Spellacy, MD, became the new chair of the department in 1988, Dr. Knupple moved on to become chairman of OB-GYN at the Robert Wood Johnson Medical School at the University of Medicine and Dentistry of New Jersey. At this point, William O'Brien, MD, a member of the division since 1983, took over the leadership of the division. Dr. O'Brien, a native of New York, was educated at Hunter College and the New York University School of Medicine. After a general medical internship at the Manhattan VA New York Harbor Healthcare Systems, he did his OB-GYN residency at Yale and his fellowship at the Bethesda Naval Hospital. He stayed on as faculty at the Uniformed Services University of the Health Sciences prior to coming to USF in 1983. With the assistance of Michael Parsons, MD—whom Dr. Spellacy brought with him from the University of Illinois–Chicago—and two recently graduated fellows, Mark Williams, MD, and Judith Krammer, MD, the division quickly grew and expanded clinical services. Ronald Chez, MD, a nationally prominent clinician and educator, was added to the division as director of ambulatory operations.

The division rapidly became the major obstetrical influence in the region. A perinatal outreach program was begun with clinics in Bartow, Dade City, New Port Richey, and Ruskin. These clinics were staffed by faculty from the division along with nurse coordinators, genetic counselors, and ultrasonographers. Two former fellows, Stephen Carlan, MD, and Timothy O'Leary, MD, after completing training, established a similar perinatal program in the Orlando area.

Even with these expanded clinical services, the division continued its research and educational mission, being the primary obstetrical teachers of USF residents and students. As mentioned, through these years, it was known as the Maternal-Fetal Medicine and Obstetrics Division, overseeing the care of all pregnant women regardless of risk. The division provided the primary impetus to open the nation's first labor-and-delivery suite made up entirely of individual labor/delivery/recovery rooms for both low-risk and high-risk obstetrical patients at Tampa General Hospital. The only LDR units to precede this were available to low-risk women only. This USF/TGH model is now the norm nationwide.

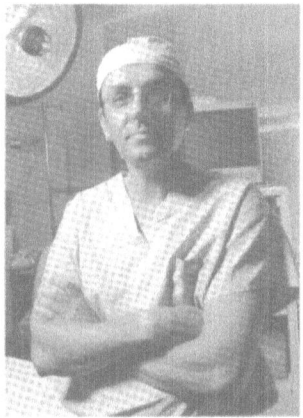

Dr. Ruben Quintero

The next step in the evolution of the division was brought about in 2005 by the addition of Ruben Quintero, MD, as division director after Dr. O'Brien entered private practice in Southwest Florida. Dr. Quintero, a native of Venezuela, came to the United States as an undergraduate student at the George Washington University. He returned to Venezuela for medical school and came back to the United States as an OB-GYN resident and MFM fellow at Yale. Dr. Quintero's international reputation in the area of fetal surgery moved the direction to a more specific consultation-oriented service with an influence far beyond Florida. The division became the center for prenatal diagnosis and treatment using advanced invasive procedures, including fetoscopy and fetal endoscopic surgery. Two new faculty, Eftichia Kontopoulos, MD, and Victoria Belogolovkin, MD, were added to this reconstituted division.

In 2009, Drs. Quintero and Kontopoulos left to join the faculty of the University of Miami and Valerie Whiteman, MD, of Temple University in Philadelphia, took on the responsibility of bringing the division into the new decade as interim director.

The Division of Reproductive Endocrinology and Infertility

by Barry S. Verkauf, MD, MBA

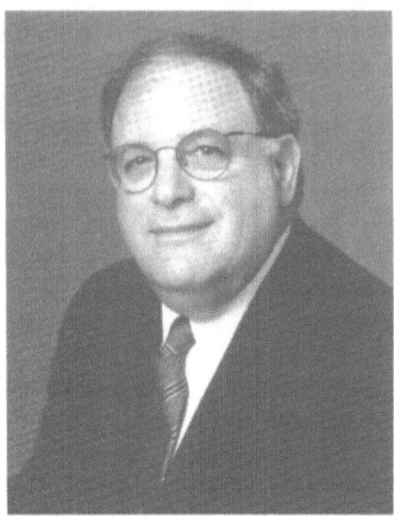

Dr. Barry S. Verkauf

Subspecialty boards were formed in 1972 for reproductive endocrinology and infertility, gynecologic oncology, and maternal-fetal medicine. Examination for special competence in these areas began in 1974. Dr. Barry S. Verkauf assumed responsibility for the Division of Reproductive Endocrinology and Infertility, having completed a fellowship with Drs. Howard and Georgeanna Jones and, on the basis of continuing responsibilities, qualified for and passed the Board Exam in Reproductive Endocrinology and Infertility. A clinic was established in this subspecialty at Tampa General Hospital for the residents to see uninsured patients at Tampa General Hospital, and private patients were seen at the clinical offices at One Davis Boulevard. In the late 1970s, Dr. Verkauf left the faculty on a full-time basis to establish one of the first private practices in infertility and reproductive endocrinology in the State of Florida. He continued to participate on a quarter-time basis as part of the medical-school faculty, administered the Midwinter Seminar, and attended the Tampa General Hospital resident REI clinic each Monday morning.

In 1981, two events coincided that significantly influenced the evolution of the division. The first was the birth of the first American child by in vitro fertilization (IVF) in Norfolk, Virginia, in the program established there by

Drs. Georgeanna and Howard Jones, who originally had gone to Norfolk to teach residents and students after their retirement from Hopkins but had started a second career in their late sixties as a consequence of their success and prominence in in vitro fertilization.

The second was the expansion of Women's Hospital, a private single-specialty facility in Tampa developed by private physicians in the community across the street from St. Joseph's Hospital. Attention during this time was turning increasingly to women's health. Privately owned hospitals, such as this one (soon owned by Humana Incorporated), were in vogue. Single-specialty OB-GYN hospitals present early in the century (e.g., Chicago Lying-In and Boston Lying-In) began to reemerge around the country and were quite successful. Humana Women's Hospital in Tampa planned to enlarge its facility and, at the suggestion of Dr. Verkauf who led an ad hoc committee created at Humana Women's Hospital to study the issue, came to the decision that it would be appropriate and possible to evolve a first-class in-vitro-fertilization program within that facility. The ad hoc committee felt that such a specialized program would require support from the entire community and would best be served by a joint community/ university undertaking. Dr. James M. Ingram, chairman of the OB-GYN Department at USF, agreed with this approach, and Dr. Verkauf took a six-week sabbatical to go to Norfolk, Virginia, to investigate the necessities of establishing a successful IVF program in Tampa. Arrangements were then made with the Department of Pediatrics for Thomas Tedesco, PhD—who directed the regional genetics program for USF—to take a year sabbatical to initiate the laboratory components of this IVF effort.

Contemporaneously with these events, having acquired a full-time director of maternal-fetal medicine and of gynecologic oncology, Dr. Ingram sought to fill the open spot of the full-time director of the Division of Reproductive Endocrinology and Infertility. Much discussion between the university and Humana Women's Hospital and its ad hoc committee took place. They agreed that the joint IVF program would be formed with a codirector from the Women's Hospital staff—which would be Dr. Verkauf, a codirector who would be the division head of reproductive endocrinology and infertility at the university—and up to six other staff physicians who would participate in the program once facilities were constructed and clinical protocols established.

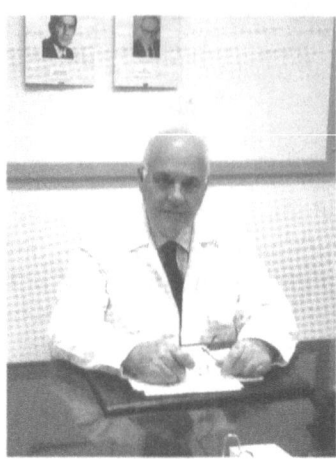

Dr. George Maroulis

During the interval when plans were being made to bring an IVF program to Tampa, discussions were being held with Dr. George B. Maroulis to be the director of the Division of Reproductive Endocrinology and Infertility. Dr. Maroulis was born in Athens, Greece, in 1940, attended precollegiate education in Athens at Athens College Preparatory School, and matriculated at Rensselaer Polytechnic Institute in Troy, New York, where he received his BS degree in biology. Four years later, in 1967, he received his doctorate in medicine from Albany Medical College. He then began a residency in obstetrics and gynecology at Duke University and subsequently became a research and clinical fellow in the Department of Obstetrics and Gynecology at UCLA David Geffen School of Medicine and at Harbor General Hospital, Division of Reproductive Biology. Having completed a two-year fellowship in that environment, he became an assistant professor at Rush Medical College and chief of the Division of Reproductive Endocrinology and Infertility. Dr. Maroulis then moved to the University of Chicago Pritzker School of Medicine, where as an associate professor, he was chief of the Division of Reproductive Endocrinology and Infertility. In 1982, he left to return to Greece, where he was chairman of the Department of Obstetrics and Gynecology at the University of Patras in Patras, Greece. Desirous of returning to the United States, he accepted the position of head of the Division of Reproductive Endocrinology at the University of South Florida in 1985.

Dr. Maroulis's arrival in the United States was delayed by an unexpected death in his family, but he and Dr. Verkauf communicated regularly by telephone. Sharing Dr. Verkauf's experience at Norfolk and with other early IVF programs in the United States and Dr. Maroulis's experience in Europe, this unique combination of a university/community combined program, despite the intensive planning required, accepted its first patient on time in January 1986. Following the advice given by the early IVF pioneers at Norfolk, the Humana/USF IVF Program remarkably achieved a pregnancy with its second patient, which turned out to be the first IVF birth in the State of Florida. This early success continued through the coordinated efforts of the radioimmunoassay laboratory, ultrasound lab, embryology lab, and andrology labs coordinated by Dr. Maroulis and Dr. Tedesco and due to the early implementation of new advances in the field

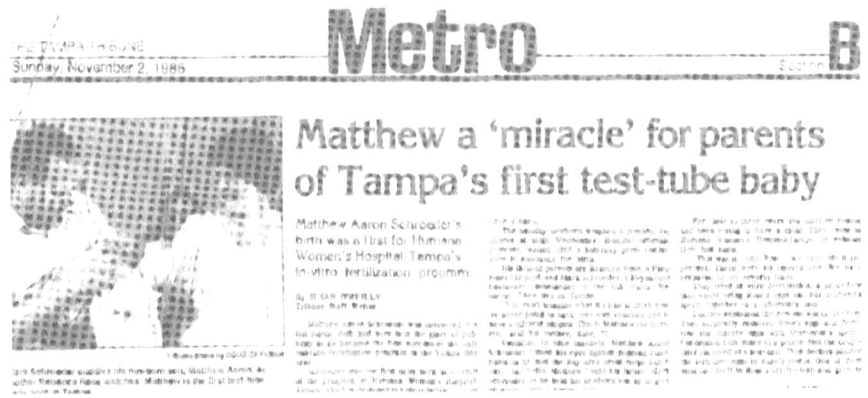

of IVF, such as transvaginal oocyte retrieval and embryo freezing. Dr. Verkauf's organizational efforts in initiating the program and Dr. Maroulis's scientific input helped ensure its early success.

In 1987, Dr. Marc Bernhisel—trained at Duke University and who had chaired the Division of Reproductive Endocrinology and Infertility at the University of Florida, had been one of its outstanding teachers, and had achieved the first gamete intrafallopian tube transfer (GIFT) pregnancy in Florida—joined Dr. Verkauf in practice and added additional expertise to the IVF group. In 1988, Dr. Timothy Yeko—who, like Dr. Bernhisel, was subspecialty boarded in reproductive endocrinology and infertility—joined the Division of Reproductive Endocrinology and Infertility at USF with Dr. Maroulis, bringing additional breadth and depth to the group. While continuing to contribute to and participate in the joint community/university IVF program based at Women's Hospital, the REI Division at USF continued to grow under the leadership of Dr. Maroulis with the help of Dr. Tim Yeko and Dr. Anna Parsons. While Dr. Parsons's interests were principally in gynecologic ultrasonography, Dr. Yeko's interests spanned the breadth of infertility and reproductive endocrinology, particularly in IVF and infertility surgery. Due to family issues, Dr. Maroulis returned to Greece to resume chairmanship of a department of obstetrics and gynecology in 1995. Dr. Yeko became chief of the Division of Reproductive Endocrinology and Infertility at USF.

Dr. Timothy R. Yeko was born in Milwaukee, educated at the University of Wisconsin undergraduate and medical schools, and completed his residency in obstetrics and gynecology at the University of Illinois in Chicago. He then did a year of fellowship at Harbor-UCLA Medical Center in Torrance, California, and a second year of fellowship at the University of Illinois in Chicago as senior research fellow in reproductive endocrinology. Dr. Yeko was always known as an excellent teacher and was recognized in this regard by students and residents alike in Chicago, Los Angeles, and at USF. A member of many professional organizations within his subspecialty, he served as an expert reviewer for all the major medical journals within his field and continued his interests in both the assisted reproductive technologies and advanced operative laparoscopy. He was principal or coinvestigator in over twenty-five research studies and has over thirty articles published in refereed journals.

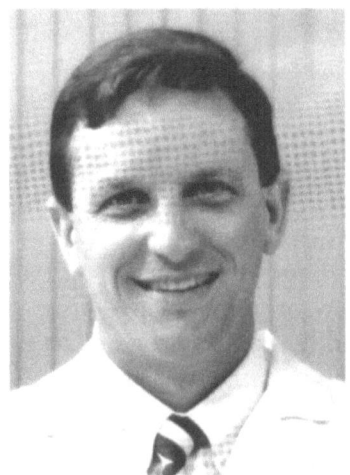

Dr. Timothy Yeko

He continued the REI fellowship started by Dr. Maroulis. The first fellow completing this track was Dr. James Mayer, who joined and remains to this day with the REI Division in the Department of Obstetrics and Gynecology. Over time, six additional fellows completed the REI fellowship at USF under Dr. Yeko's direction. Drs. Petty Zourepolis, Pak Chung, Gerald

Natovsky, Marcello Barrionueva, Anna Nackley, and Mark Sanchez have all found successful niches within the field of reproductive endocrinology at various academic and private practices around the country.

In 1995, further changes occurred within the division. In addition to the loss of Dr. Maroulis to Greece, Humana Women's Hospital was purchased by St. Joseph's Hospital, a Catholic institution, and the IVF program was unable to remain in that facility. Drs. Verkauf and Bernhisel moved their IVF efforts to Florida Hospital Tampa and joined with Dr. Samuel Tarantino in what became the Reproductive Medicine Group. After a brief time at Tampa Outpatient Surgical Facility, the USF Division of Reproductive Endocrinology and Infertility (REI) efforts in IVF came under the rubric of the Center for Human Reproduction, whose corporate headquarters were in Chicago. Dr. Yeko was the Florida director of the Center for Human Reproduction (CHR). He recruited Dr. Alice Rhoton-Vlasak from the University of Florida to assist him and Dr. James Mayer in this effort. Dr. Rhoton-Vlasak subsequently returned to the University of Florida. In 2000, Dr. Yeko joined the Reproductive Medicine Group with Drs. Verkauf, Bernhisel, Tarantino, and Goodman. He continued to head the Division of Reproductive Endocrinology and Infertility at USF on a part-time basis. As a consequence, students and residents had exposure within the environment of private medicine as well as academic medicine in reproductive endocrinology and infertility, and they continued to score high on their testing in this subspecialty. This arrangement continued until the arrival of Dr. Shayne Plosker in 2006.

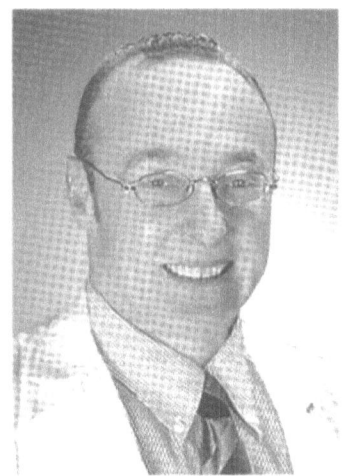

Dr. Shayne Plosker

Dr. Shayne Plosker came to Tampa with the unique background of having been in both academic medicine and private practice. He was born in Canada, did his undergraduate training at University of Western Ontario and the University of Manitoba and completed medical school at the University of Western Ontario and his residency there in obstetrics and gynecology in 1987. He then completed a fellowship in reproductive endocrinology and infertility at the University of California, San Francisco. He was an attending physician at Toronto General Hospital and assistant professor at the University of Toronto until he moved to Falls River, Massachusetts, where he was in active private practice of REI for ten years before being recruited to join the Division of Reproductive Endocrinology and Infertility at Brown University Alpert Medical School in 2002. While at Toronto General, as well as at Brown University, he was regularly recognized by the faculty, resident staff, and students as an outstanding teacher. At Brown, he coordinated the donor-egg program and was actively involved in IVF, both at Brown University and at Tufts University with Dr. David Keefe and Ying Ying, PhD. After Dr. Keefe accepted the chairmanship of the Department of OB-GYN at USF in Tampa, he asked both Drs. Plosker and Ying to join him, which they did in 2006.

At that time, there was no IVF program unique to the Department of Obstetrics and Gynecology. With the support and help of Dr. Keefe, Dr. Plosker initiated a new program to be located at Tampa General Hospital, not only providing general IVF and ART services, but with a specific focus on unique facets that would complement what was already in the community. With the Department of Genetics, a preimplantation genetics program and a gestational surrogacy program were initiated, and a serious commitment was made with Tampa's Moffitt Cancer Center for a fertility-preservation program to provide embryo-, sperm-, and egg-freezing capability for young women and young men with cancer. The Livestrong Foundation had recognized Moffitt and the USF IVF program as a center of excellence for care of these unfortunate couples.

The success of the IVF program generated increased interest in establishing a women's care center at Tampa General Hospital to more broadly meet the needs of women's health in a newly constructed environment in which the IVF laboratory, operating rooms, and research facilities are now housed.

Research interests within the division have focused around egg maturation, improving vitrification techniques, embryo and egg freezing, and fertility preservation. Dr. Celso Silva joined the department in 2007 with a K30 scholar NIH grant to receive a master's in translational research and has been the director of the fertility preservation program since his arrival.

Student and resident teaching within the division has continued to emphasize collaboration with the section on pediatric endocrinology in addition to the breadth of disorders in reproductive physiology in women from birth into adolescence and through menopause.

The Division of General Obstetrics and Gynecology

by *Catherine Lynch, MD*

Most clinical academic departments in the United States developed as tertiary-care centers focusing on subspecialty care. This was true of obstetrics and gynecology as well as other medical and surgical specialties. By the mid-1990s, Dr. Spellacy clearly saw a need to develop a Division of General Obstetrics and Gynecology to complement the divisions of reproductive endocrinology and infertility, gynecologic oncology, and maternal-fetal medicine, which already existed. The purpose of the division was not only to provide medical students and residents with exposure to what practice as a generalist now entailed, but also to generate a clinical patient base that would also help sustain the subspecialists by referrals.

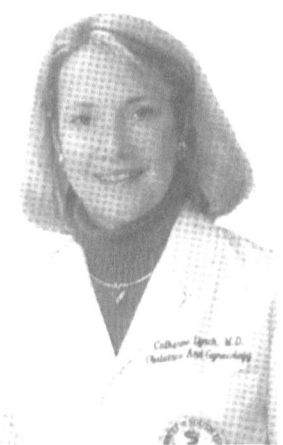

Dr. Catherine Lynch

In 1997, the Division of General Obstetrics and Gynecology was created and Dr. Catherine Lynch was appointed the division director. Dr. Lynch was raised in Florida. She received her BS degree in biology from Georgetown University and was planning to stay there for medical school when she interviewed at the University of South Florida. Much to her surprise, she was struck by the city that Tampa had become and impressed by people at the medical school and in town who reminded her of the "old Floridians" with whom she had grown up. Thus, she returned to Florida to attend USF. At the start of her third year of medical school, Dr. William Spellacy arrived to head the Department of Obstetrics and Gynecology. Dr. Lynch was an outstanding student and was selected for Alpha Omega Alpha Honor Medical Society. After interviewing for residency at top programs around the country, she became certain that USF was the right fit for her residency.

Early in Dr. Lynch's fourth year of residency, Dr. Spellacy pulled her aside one day as they were working together on labor and delivery. He asked her if she would like to join the department as a generalist and have the opportunity to develop an area of special interest. In 1994, Dr. Lynch joined the department, practicing general obstetrics and gynecology in the Division of Gynecology. Dr. Lynch developed a focus in urogynecology at the Bay Pines Veterans Administration (VA) Healthcare System. Through this patient experience—as well as additional educational opportunities, including going to Boston to shadow Dr. David Nichols—she continued to expand her knowledge in urogynecology. Her experience at the Bay Pines VA, in addition to Tampa General, gave her over 160 *gyn* cases in one year to demonstrate when she applied for her oral boards. She continued the urogynecology service, which had been established at Bay Pines, and instituted urodynamic studies both at Bay Pines and at Harbourside departmental office in Tampa.

In 1995, Dr. L. Amy Boardman joined the department from the University of South Florida as a generalist. Dr. Boardman was also originally from Florida, raised in Winter Park. Drs. Boardman and Lynch started building a "private" obstetric practice within the OB-GYN department and cross-covered for each other for deliveries. Shortly after Dr. Boardman joined the faculty, the James A. Haley Veterans' Hospital in Tampa decided to expand their gynecology services, and Dr. Boardman spent part of her time at the Haley Veterans' Hospital. Both the practices of Dr. Lynch and Dr. Boardman continued to grow, but the need for further expansion was recognized.

The Division of General Obstetrics and Gynecology was formed by Dr. Spellacy in 1997 when Dr. Angela Keating joined the department, forming a nucleus of three OB-GYN generalists. Dr. Keating completed her residency at the University of Cincinnati. Dr. Lynch turned over the Bay Pines VA clinics to Dr. Keating and began to focus her own attention full-time to the growth of the new Division of Obstetrics and Gynecology and its practice. The next year, Dr. Lorraine Bevilacqua came from Pittsburgh to join the division; her husband, Dr. Raoul Salup, had been recruited by the

Department of Urology. Drs. Lynch, Boardman, Keating, and Bevilacqua continued to build the practice of general obstetrics and gynecology within the department. Dr. Lynch continued her interest in urogynecology as well.

The millennium was tumultuous for the division, with many changes that were related to their being an all-woman group. Dr. Bevilacqua, who had come from private practice at Magee-Womens Hospital in Pittsburgh, decided to take an opportunity with a private-practice group in Tampa. Dr. Boardman had her first child, and both Drs. Lynch and Keating became married. Dr. Boardman's husband, a PhD in psychology, took an opportunity in Greenville, South Carolina, and she moved there with him. Dr. Keating's husband, a civil engineer, was transferred to Panama City, Florida, and she accompanied him. Fortunately, Dr. Joan McCarthy joined the division after completing her residency at USF. Dr. Karen Bruder left the faculty at Eastern Virginia Medical School and came to Tampa to take over the medical directorship of Genesis. Dr. Lauri Hochberg also joined the division, having come to Tampa with her husband, David, a urologist who joined his father's practice.

The reconstituted Division of General Obstetrics and Gynecology continued to build over the next several years. Dr. Carol Cox joined the division while her husband, John, completed his residency training in general surgery. After her husband decided to establish his practice in Tampa, Dr. Cox has remained in the department and has been instrumental in the growth of the division at the USF campus site in North Tampa. Dr. Shelly Holmstrom came to Tampa with her husband, Bjorn, after training in Savanna. Dr. Holmstrom likes to point out that while she interviewed at USF for medical school and residency, she was only accepted when interviewed for a faculty position. Dr. Holmstrom has become a leader in medical-student education and is the course director of the maternal/newborn clerkship.

Over the next several years, the division grew with the addition of Drs. Marissa Baker, Christine Tebes, Maggie Keloing, Kelly Hamel, and Amanda Avelo-Malina. These young, enthusiastic generalists were important in allowing the division to provide service to patients who had no attending physician at Florida Hospital Tampa (FHT) as well as at Tampa General Hospital. Concurrent with the contract for coverage with FHT was an agreement to assume physician coverage for the midwives of Women's Health Center who practiced at Tampa General Hospital. With that agreement, Dr. J. Donald Burgess joined the division, bringing his twenty-five years of clinical experience into the group.

It became quite clear with the increase in responsibilities for coverage noted above, as well as the continued growth of the private practice, that additional providers focused principally on seeing private patients were needed. Dr. Sheila Connery, after twenty years of solo practice in Rhode Island, decided to follow Dr. Keefe when he became chairman and joined the division. At this time, it became clear that the division would need to accommodate and maximize each member's strengths and interests. A delineation was made between the activities of those focused on growth of the private practice and those with more of an active role at Genesis and a resident and medical student education. Dr. Erich Wykoff, trained at Wright State University, joined the group from a federally funded health department center in Manatee County. His focus was on minimally invasive surgery. Dr. Susan Smith, having completed her training at USF, also joined with the desire to build an academic generalist practice.

A key addition to the division, Dr. Jim Palmer, broadened its focus to include the development of research-oriented academic generalists. After completing his residency at USF, Dr. Palmer joined the division with a part-time clinical appointment and part-time academic appointment to strengthen his résumé in research. In that initial two years, he completed a master's in medical research (MMR) and was a member of the K30 program. His administrative abilities became evident, and he was appointed the assistant residency-program director under Dr. Spellacy.

The generalist division has continued to develop and take on new responsibilities since its founding in 1997. It is now the economic engine of the department, not only fueling patient referrals to subspecialties, but also providing the financial support for the department to continue to develop outstanding research and maintain its educational mission. Future plans include offering an academic generalist "fellowship" in which individuals completing their residency training will be able to spend part of their time getting either a master's of science or master's of public health while further developing their clinical and educational skills. This is designed to enrich the breadth and depth of not only the Division of General Obstetrics and Gynecology, but the entire department as well.

The Division of Gynecologic Specialties

by J. K. Williams, MD

When Dr. Michael Parsons took over as interim chair in 2002, his vision was to evolve the Division of Gynecology into the Division of Gynecologic Specialties. He recognized that specific areas of gynecologic care in an academic center needed to expand beyond the traditional roles of general gynecology, gynecologic oncology, and reproductive endocrinology/infertility.

Dr. J. K. Williams led this "new" division, having been previously the director of the Division of Gynecology.

Dr. Williams was raised in Detroit, educated at the University of Michigan, and trained at Wayne State University. He first joined the faculty at Wayne State University in 1978 after approximately three years in a busy private practice. In 1982, Dr. Ingram recruited him to join the USF faculty as director of the residency program, a position he held until 1988. In 1985, he was named the outstanding residency-program director in ACOG's District IV. Interestingly, Dr. Williams's original academic interest was in obstetrics, having been one of the first maternal-fetal medicine fellows in the department and having served as clinical administrator for obstetrical services for Tampa General Hospital from 1985 to1988. However, having never lost interest in gynecology, Dr. Williams became the director of the Division of Gynecology upon the death of Dr. Ingram in 1989.

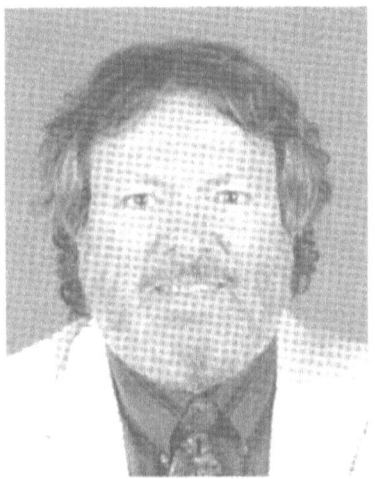

Dr. J. K. Williams

The divisions rapidly sprang forth, the first being gynecologic ultrasound headed by Dr. Anna Parsons. With the continuing support of the next department chairman, Dr. David Keefe, the divisions of urogynecology/pelvic reconstructive surgery, directed by Dr. Lennox Hoyte; minimally invasive gynecologic surgery, directed by Dr. Larry Glazerman; and chronic pelvic pain, directed by Dr. Gerard DiLeo, came into being. The detailed history of these divisions follows.

The Division of Urogynecology

by *Lennox Hoyte, MD, MSEE*

Procedures to address pelvic organ prolapse and urinary incontinence have been performed by members of the USF OB-GYN group for many years. Dr. Catherine Lynch was an early provider of urogynecologic services for the USF OB-GYN group and purchased the first urodynamics testing machine for the department.

A formal division of female pelvic medicine and reconstructive surgery was started in 2006, with the hiring of Lennox Hoyte, MD. With a master's in engineering and computer science from MIT, obstetric and gynecologic training at Harvard, and a fellowship in female pelvic medicine

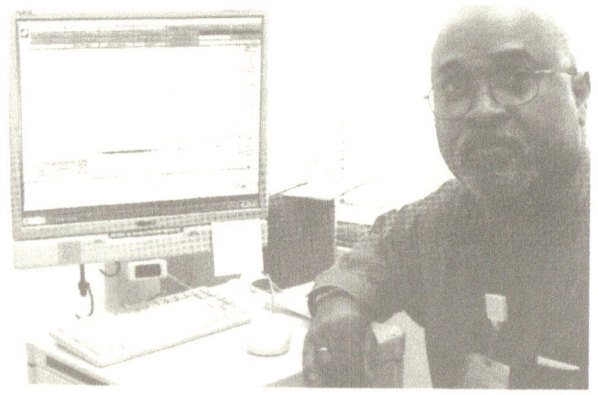

Dr. Lennox Hoyte

and reconstructive surgery from Loyola University, Dr. Hoyte developed the multidisciplinary pelvic-floor-disorders group at Tampa General Hospital, our partner hospital. The Pelvic Floor Disorders Group includes specialists from colorectal surgery, urology, physical therapy, gynecologic imaging, and psychology. Together, the group evaluates and treats complex cases of female pelvic-floor dysfunction. The division added Dr. Stuart Hart, a fellowship-trained pelvic surgeon and expert laparoscopist. Together, Drs. Hoyte and Hart see and treat women with complex pelvic-floor disorders, including prolapse, urinary and fecal incontinence, bladder-control problems, and pelvic and bladder pain, as well as fistulas related to the urinary, reproductive, and gastrointestinal tracts. Complex multichannel urodynamic testing and office cystoscopy procedures are offered at the Tampa location. The division performs over six hundred surgical procedures annually, primarily at Tampa General Hospital. Formal application for fellowship status has recently been approved. The division added a nurse practitioner, Leigh Terwilliger, in 2009. Today, the urogynecology group is a leading center for robotic and laparoscopic urogynecology procedures as well as transvaginal and open approaches for treating all types of female pelvic-floor disorders.

The Urogynecology Division is active in clinical research related to pelvic-floor disorders, with a focus on pelvic-floor imaging and biomechanics.

The Division of Gynecologic Imaging

by *Barry S. Verkauf, MD, MBA*

Leonardo da Vinci was the first to attempt to detect sound waves underwater during the fifteenth century,[1] but it wasn't until World Wars I and II that sound waves (*sonar*) were used as a technique of locating, imaging, and determining the size of and distance of vessels in water. During the early 1960s, high frequency sound waves (ultrasound) were used in England in obstetrical care, and in the late 1960s, use began in the United States for the purpose principally of placental localization, excluding placenta previa and abruption. Since that time, the use of ultrasound in both obstetrics and gynecology has become extraordinarily widespread.

Dr. Anna Parsons trained in both obstetrics and gynecology and reproductive endocrinology at the University of Illinois in Chicago. After serving one year as an assistant professor in that department, she moved to Tampa to join her former mentor, Dr. Spellacy, and to initiate an image-based gynecology clinic. Dr. Parsons has authored over twenty-five peer-reviewed articles and contributed to twelve chapters in textbooks. She is a member of the International Society of Ultrasound in Obstetrics and Gynecology and served on its governing board from 1999 to 2005. She also is a fellow of the American Institute of Ultrasound in Medicine, as well as the American Congress of Obstetricians and Gynecologists. She has served as a reviewer for virtually every major obstetric and gynecologic journal in this country and has received eighteen grants relative to the use of ultrasound and studying the impact of various hormones—such as estrogen, MPA, tibolone, and raloxifene—on the endometrium.

Dr. Parsons currently is an associate professor of obstetrics and gynecology and the director of the image-based gynecology clinic at USF.

---

[1] Frank Fahy and John Bernard Walker, eds, *Fundamentals of Noise and Vibrations* (Taylor & Francis), 375.

She has contributed to notable advances in the field (including the use of the Tampa catheter to facilitate the use of saline-infusion sonography for detection of uterine intracavitary defects), is investigating the use of ionic solutions used transcervically and monitored sonographically to avoid the use of iodizing radiation in hysterosalpingography, and has been among the first to investigate the use of three-dimensional and four-dimensional ultrasound.

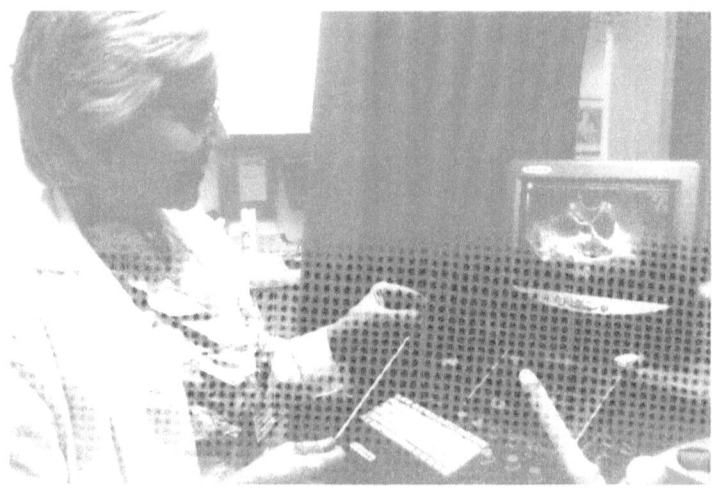

Dr. Anna Parsons

Dr. Parsons uses diagnostic imaging for a wide variety of purposes and is currently involved in interdisciplinary research with the Division of Pelvic Medicine, providing image-based guidance for their surgical procedures.

The Division of Image-Based Gynecology provides extensive clinical services within the department for all divisions and receives referrals from the nonuniversity community. In 1997, Dr. Parsons was joined by Dr. Lori Hochberg, increasing the research capacity and clinical capacity of the image-based gynecology clinic.

The Division of Minimally Invasive Gynecologic Surgery

by Larry Glazerman, MD, MBA

Members of the OB-GYN Department at USF have been performing minimally invasive procedures for decades, including diagnostic laparoscopy and hysteroscopy as well as laparoscopic tubal sterilizations. While gynecologists developed laparoscopy in the 1950s, the technique exploded in the 1980s with the advent of laparoscopic cholecystectomy performed by general-surgical colleagues.

The first laparoscopic hysterectomies were performed nationally in the 1980s. Members of this department started performing laparoscopic-assisted vaginal hysterectomies in the 1990s. In contrast to the general surgeons, OB-GYN specialists have been slow to adopt minimally invasive techniques for hysterectomy; only about 15 percent of hysterectomies nationally are performed laparoscopically, with another 20 percent being done vaginally and 65 percent performed by the traditional open-abdominal route.

Recognizing this disparity, Dr. Keefe, in conjunction with Dr. Klasko, recruited Dr. Larry Glazerman to the department in 2008 to establish a formal division of minimally invasive gynecologic surgery. Dr. Glazerman is nationally and internationally recognized as a leader in the area, serving on the board of the International Society for Gynecologic Endoscopy, as well as many other professional societies. Dr. Glazerman, in collaboration with Dr. Stuart Hart of the Division of Urogynecology and Dr. Deborah Sutherland of the Office of Continuing Professional Development, instituted the Center for Advancement of Minimally-Invasive Pelvic Surgery (CAMPS). The center is charged with training medical students, residents, and practicing physicians through continuing-medical-education courses. As part of their third-year gyn surgery rotation, medical students spend a session in the USF Center for Advanced Medical Learning and Simulation at Tampa General Hospital, working on both laparoscopic and hysteroscopic simulators. The simulation center at TGH was the first center in the country to obtain the HystSim™ virtual-reality hysteroscopic simulator, manufactured by VirtaMed AG in Zurich, Switzerland. In the summer of 2010, Drs. Glazerman and Hart, as principal investigators in conjunction with Simbionix—an Israeli manufacturer of surgical simulators—were awarded a $700,000 grant by the Binational Industrial Research and Development (BIRD) Foundation, a joint venture of the Israeli and US governments, which sponsors cooperative ventures between US and Israeli companies. This was only the second BIRD grant awarded to an academic institution and will result in a laparoscopic hysterectomy module for the Simbionix Lap Mentor virtual-reality laparoscopic simulator.

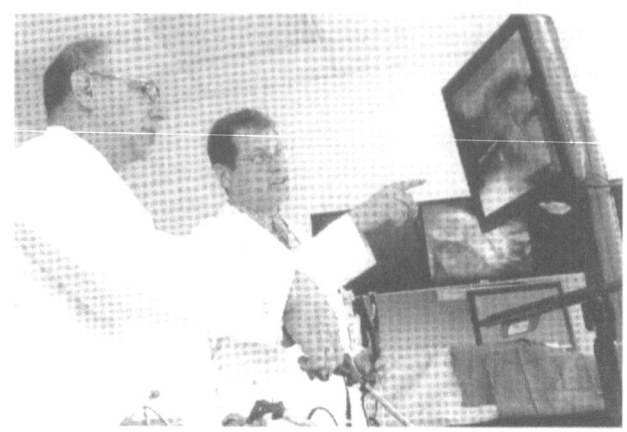

Drs. Larry Glazerman and Stuart Hart

In addition, the Division of Minimally Invasive GYN Surgery has been in the forefront of training and clinical care with the da Vinci Surgical System, both at Tampa General Hospital and the USF Health da Vinci Center for Computer Assisted Surgery. Dr. Glazerman has performed over one hundred procedures using the da Vinci system in addition to traditional laparoscopic and hysteroscopic procedures. Starting with the 2010–2011 academic year, a formal curriculum was instituted to train residents in minimally invasive surgery, including certification in fundamentals of laparoscopic surgery. Plans are underway for a fellowship in minimally invasive gynecologic surgery as well, sponsored by the American Association of Gynecologic Laparoscopists.

The Division of Gynecologic Research

by John Tsibris, PhD

The Research Division was established as a separate administrative unit of the department when Dr. Spellacy became chairman in 1988.

Its first member and director was John C. M. Tsibris, PhD, who had worked for Dr. Spellacy at the University of Miami, University of Florida, and University of Illinois. Upon his arrival, he set up wet-chemistry laboratories in a 3,600 sq. ft. area allotted by Tampa General Hospital on the ground floor of the east wing. State-of-the-art equipment for a mini biochemistry department was purchased, and two more faculty members joined the division two years later, Mark P. McLean, PhD, and Jeanne L. Becker, PhD.

Easy access to surgical specimens, from the Tampa General Hospital operating rooms and labor-and-delivery suites, was a great catalyst for basic research of human tissues. These laboratories were especially efficient and convenient for OB-GYN residents, maternal-fetal-medicine (MFM) fellows, reproductive endocrinology and infertility (REI) fellows, gynecologic-oncology fellows, postdoctoral fellows, and medical and premedical students who were interested in research, as well as trainee physicians from China, Japan, and the Republic of Georgia.

Amicable collaborations soon developed with research teams under Papineni S. Rao, PhD, from the Gynecologic Oncology Division and William F. O'Brien, MD, and Kathy B. Porter, MD, from the MFM Division, who were engaged in basic research at the OB-GYN laboratories and the excellent surgical suite for animal-model work located in the "north" college of medicine campus on Bruce B. Downs Boulevard.

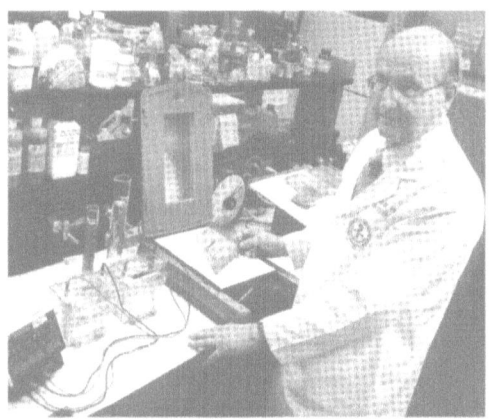

Dr. John Tsibris

In 2003, Tampa General Hospital reassigned the Research Division's laboratory space that was relocated to the north campus. Human-tissue acquisition became less convenient, but proximity to the newly established (first in the State of Florida) core laboratories for microarrays, proteomics, and cell imaging at the Moffitt Cancer Center and to the USF vivarium facilitated work and opened new avenues for research.

In 2006, the arrival of the new OB-GYN chair, Dr. David L. Keefe, his close associate, Lin Liu, PhD, and later, Celso Silva, MD, enriched research with innovative technologies—such as those in stem-cell research—and an influx of physician trainees, graduate students, and faculty collaborators from Brazil and China.

The division's research agenda is well established. To date, over four hundred articles emanating from the obstetrics-and-gynecology department have been published, many with OB-GYN research funds, and later supported by federal, state, and pharmaceutical grants. Detailed information on published articles from these collaborations can be obtained by searching PubMed.

A few highlights of the research in the Research Division's laboratories with OB-GYN and other USF and national and international collaborators are as follows:

- *Primary breast-carcinoma growth in three-dimensional cultures and inhibition by aspirin of ovarian-tumor-cell growth (Becker).* Some of her research was supported by NASA, and her cultures were tested by NASA in space.

- *Regulation of HDL receptor by estrogens and steroidogenic proteins (McLean).* He received twice (a first for USF) the American Heart Association's Robert J. Boucek Research Merit Award (1993, 2001) and the Society for Gynecologic Investigation (SGI) President's Award in 1992. He has been supported with five NIH grants ($7.5 million), six American Heart grants ($800,000), and two grants from the Florida Department of Health with colleagues from OB-GYN (Liu and Keefe) and the Biochemistry Department ($1.2 million). He has published thirty-five peer-review papers and fifty-five abstracts at USF.

- *Postdoctoral research associates (Rosalyn Irby and Dayami Lopez) were supported by American Heart Association Fellowships and Development Award (Dayami Lopez).* Todd Sandhoff, graduate student and later postdoctoral fellow, received the Study of Reproduction New Investigator Award in 1997. Pak Chung, REI fellow, received a fellowship from the Florida Society of Reproductive Endocrinology and the SGI President's Presenter's Award in 1997. Anna Nackley, REI fellow, received the President of the SGI Presenter's Award in 2000 and 2001, and SGI's Blue Ribbon Presentation Recognition in 2000.

- *The first human-genome screening by mRNA arrays of human fibroids revealed new angiogenesis genes (Tsibris et al.).* A guinea-pig model was developed for fibroids of the uterus (Tsibris, Porter, O'Brien et al.) and received a US patent; the effect of vitamin-D receptor agonists on leiomyoma development was studied in the model (Tsibris, supported by BioXell, Milan).

- *Umbilical plasma erythropoietin, a marker of fetal hypoxia, in a series of six peer-reviewed papers by maternal-fetal-medicine fellow Allahyar Jazayeri, Spellacy, Tsibris et al.*
- *Prostaglandin-E receptors, interleukins, and preterm labor (Eric Spaziani, O'Brien, Tsibris, et al.).* A $5,000 prize was awarded by the editors of *Obstetrics & Gynecology* as one of the four outstanding manuscripts published in this journal in 1999.
- *Telomere length and pluripotency of stem cells and telomere susceptibility to cigarette-smoke-induced chromosomal instability in mouse embryos (Junjiu Huang, Liu, Keefe et al., supported by the Esther King Biomedical Research Program) were published in* Stem Cells, Nature Cell Biology, *and* Nature.

The Department of Obstetrics and Gynecology had one of the strongest clinical research programs in the USF Morsani College of Medicine in the 1980s and '90s. While there were some investigator-initiated projects, the majority of studies were sponsored by the pharmaceutical industry (e.g., antibiotic use in obstetrics and hormone therapy in gynecology). Recently, the pharmaceutical and medical instrumentation industries have come under increased scrutiny and regulation relative to investigative projects. Currently, there have been more investigator-initiative projects within the department facilitated by research coordinator Caroline Young, RN. The number has increased rapidly in recent times due to the greater number of specialties within the department and greater emphasis on research. A research committee was formed in 2010 to help foster the interest of young investigators and review their progress before their presentation to the investigational review board in hopes of stimulating innovative ideas and shortening the time and effort in bringing them to realization.

Research becomes an increasingly emphasized domain in the Department of Obstetrics and Gynecology, and the Division of Research remains active and vibrant today.

Chronic Pelvic Pain

by *Gerard M. DiLeo, MD*

Chronic pelvic pain, like all chronic pain, is a very difficult condition to treat. Typical protocols used for nonpelvic pain do not easily jump specialty lines to women's health care. In 2006, to bridge this gap, under the vision and direction of Gerard M. DiLeo, the USF Department of Obstetrics and Gynecology began the Chronic Pelvic Pain Clinic. Partnering with

———

the Division of Minimally Invasive Gynecological Surgery, the Ultrasound Imaging Clinic, and the Urogynecology Division, a centralized source for evaluation and therapy for these troubled, sometimes hopeless patients was established. Such a clinic is rare, and USF led the Southeast in instituting this much needed direction in women's health care.

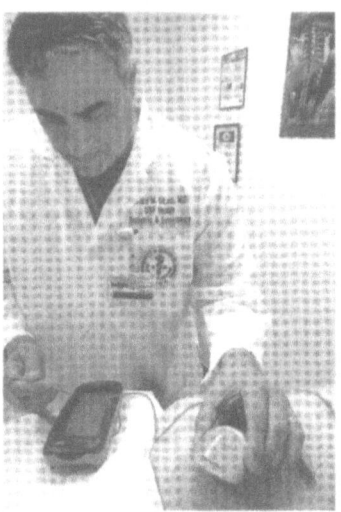

Gerard M. DiLeo, MD

Comorbidities are common. The interrelationship among fibromyalgia, migraines, TMJ dysfunction, IBS, painful bladder syndrome, and sexual abuse are addressed. The Chronic Pelvic Pain Clinic serves as an air-traffic control tower of sorts. Patients are not lost to follow-up by being sent on a linear series of endless consultations.

Besides making prudent use of an organized team approach, the Chronic Pelvic Pain Clinic also seeks to implement novel therapies that have proven efficacious above the waist. The use of intrathecal pumps to deliver microdoses of muscle relaxant affords the opportunity to provide relief without worries of side effects, addition, tolerance, or withdrawal. They have been useful in treating pelvic pain originating from pelvic-floor dysfunction and spasm, the most common feature in patients with chronic pelvic pain. Also, well established in the chronic-pain world is the technique of neurostimulation for neuropathic pain—the other common feature of pelvic pain, which often exists in a vicious positive-feedback loop with pelvic-floor muscle spasm. Both topical neurostimulation in the clinic setting as well as implanted epidural neurostimulation electrodes have made a huge impact on patients who have found themselves at a dead end of what is traditionally offered. Even vulvodynia has been treated successfully using these techniques.

Making use of traditionally nongynecological techniques, such as neurostimulation and· implantable intrathecal pumps, is only one aspect of the chronic-pain approach to chronic pelvic pain. Rational polypharmacology, including the use of neuromodulators, the newer antidepressants which also impact pain (the SSRI/NRIs), and Botox therapy for downregulating nociceptors, have complemented the mechanical and electrical approaches in treating pelvic pain.

Dr. Dileo subsequently entered private practice in West Central Florida.

Table 11

Clinical Subspecialty Division—Directors and Fellows

Division of Gynecologic Oncology

Division Directors

Denis Cavanagh, MD	1978–1999
Mitchel Hoffman, MD	1999–present

Past/Current Fellows	Completion Date
John Shepherd, MD	1981
Donald Marsden, MD	1984
S. C. Peter Bryson, MD	1986
Mitchel Hoffman, MD	1987
James Fiorica, MD	1989
Desmond P. J. Barton, MD	1991
Noreen Gleeson, MD	1993
James Mark, MD	1994
Donna Pinelli, MD	1996
Steven DeCesare, MD	1996
Hector Arango, MD	1997
Janet Drake, MD	1999
John Bomalaski, MD	1999
John Durfee, MD	2000
Richard Cardosi, MD	2002

Katie Wakeley, MD	2002
David Griffin, MD	2003
Martin Martino, MD	2005
Brenda Shoup, MD	2005
Robyn Sayer, MD	2006
Stephen Tebes, MD	2006
Megan Indermaur, MD	2009
Marcia Humphrey, MD	2010
Nish Bansal, MD	2011
Hye Sook Chon, MD	2012
Xiaomang Stickles, MD	2013
Nadim Bou Zgheib, MD	2014

Division of Reproductive Endocrinology

REI Division Directors

Barry S. Verkauf, MD, MBA	1974–85
George Maroulis, MD	1985–96
Timothy Yeko, MD	1996–2005
Shayne Plosker, MD	2006–present

Past/Current Fellows	Completion Date
James Mayer, MD	1994
Petty Zourepolis, MD	1995
Pak Chung, MD	1996
Marcello Barioneuva, MD	1997
Jeryl Natovsky, MD	1998
Anna Nackley, MD	1999
Mark Sanchez, MD	2000

Division of Maternal-Fetal Medicine

MFM Division Directors

Robert A. Knuppel, MD, MPH	1979–89
William F. O'Brien, MD	1989–2003

William Spellacy, MD	2003–2005
Ruben Quintero, MD	2005–2009
Valerie Whiteman, MD	2009–present

Past/Current Fellows	Completion Date
Dinesh M. Shah, MD	1983
Pawan Rattan, MD	1984
Raul Montenegro, MD	1984
J. Kell Williams, MD	1985
Jeffrey Angel, MD	1986
Gary Cohen, MD	1986
Walter Morales, MD	1988
Cynthia Sims, MD	1989
Mark C. Williams, MD	1989
Marcello Pietrantoni, MD	1990
Stephen Carlan, MD	1990
Dimitrios Mastrogiannis, MD	1991
Shirley K. Sawai, MD	1991
Judith Krammer, MD	1992
James Pendergraft III, MD	1993
Timothy O'Leary, MD	1993
Alfredo Rodriguez, MD	1993
Craig Kalter, MD	1994
Armando Fuentes, MD	1994
Michael Lantz, MD	1995
John Busowski, MD	1995
Allahyar Jazayeri, MD	1998
David C. Gore, MD	2001
Adam C. Urato, MD	2003
Julie Platt, MD	2003
Jose Hernandez-Robles, MD	2006
Alan Neuman, MD	2007
Zoi Russell, MD	2008
Kimberly Destefano, MD	2009
Aaron B. Deutsch, MD	2010
Luminita Crisan, MD	2011
Kiran Rao, MD	2012

Division of Urogynecology and Pelvic Reconstructive Surgery

Division Directors

| Lennox Hoyte MD | 2006–present |

Past/Current Fellows	Completion Date
Renee Bassaly	2012
Mona McCullough	2013
Kristie Green	2014

Division of Minimally Invasive Gynecologic Surgery

Division Directors

| Larry Glazerman | 2010–2012 |
| Stuart Hart | 2012–present |

Past/Current Fellows	Completion Date
Marc Zacharius	2013

Introduction to Chapter 6

The Times, They Are a Changin'

Entrepreneurs are risk takers who engage in new enterprises, ventures, or ideas and assume accountability for their outcomes. When times and societal structure are stable, entrepreneurial activity is low. Entrepreneurs are more visible during times of (or which they perceive as) opportunity. Opportunity is present generally during unsettled times or during times of crisis.

By 2005, while not in crisis, circumstances of the medical profession were clearly unsettled and in flux. Most physicians were captive to contractual relationships with managed-care companies in order to survive. Not only had they lost their autonomy, but they had lost the opportunity to fairly set their value in an open marketplace. Physician reimbursements were established by managed-care companies, rarely negotiable, and increasingly consistent with the low reimbursements by Medicare. In turn, Medicare reimbursements were set by the sustainable growth formula (SGF), originated by Congress in 1997, which early on came to be seen as flawed and unworkable. Yet yearly, Congress failed to correct it. Physician income was declining.

In addition, the burden of paperwork required of physicians to comply with managed-care contracts was becoming untenable, given that each managed-care organization had its own forms and processes to be followed. This required more office staff, adding to the cost of practicing medicine.

In addition to burgeoning office expenses from personnel, professional liability (malpractice) premiums were skyrocketing—becoming unaffordable for some physicians in high-risk specialties. The risk of medical liability caused physicians to order more tests, thus further increasing the cost burden of medical care. Technological advances further increased medical costs, as did the increasing number of geriatric patients with multiple comorbidities.

To protect their profit margins, insurance companies continually increase their premiums, thereby increasing costs to businesses, which (of necessity) competing in a new global economy, pass the costs down to the employee and consumer.

By this time, while the majority of employed Americans were insured (though not without economic stress) by their employer, over half of Americans were covered by government programs—principally Medicare and Medicaid, where increasing cost burdens were felt as well. Fifteen percent of Americans were uninsured by virtue of being out of work, not eligible for government programs, or through their own choice. Their medical costs, when they occurred, were absorbed into and reflected by the premium costs of the privately insured.

The hospital was once described as "the physician's workshop." Physician and hospital interests had always been aligned, but in this environment, in order to reduce patient costs and capture additional income, physicians increasingly brought procedures previously done in the hospital to outside imaging centers, outpatient surgery facilities, or into their own offices or office laboratories. Hospitals began to buy physician practices. The alignment between physician and hospital interests began to diverge.

The sustainability of medical practice increasingly came to depend upon business efficiency in addition to the standard goals and measures of patient satisfaction and good medical outcomes. The symbiotic structure that formerly existed between physicians, patients, hospitals, and insurance companies and government began to quake and show signs of crumbling. Enter entrepreneurship. Entrepreneurs emerge from the population on demand due to the combination of opportunities and people well positioned with the vision and creative and innovative skills to take advantage of them.

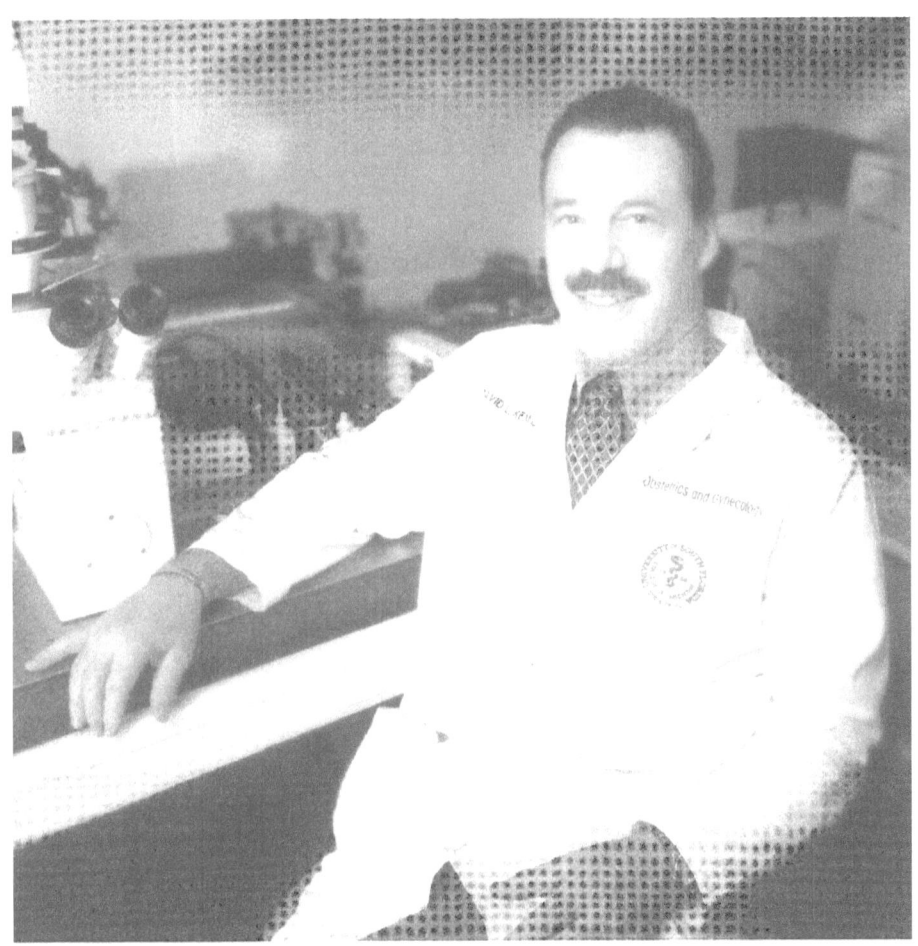

Dr. David L. Keefe

CHAPTER 6

Dr. David L. Keefe

by Shayne Plosker, MD

David L. Keefe, MD, became the third permanent chairman of the USF Department of Obstetrics and Gynecology in late 2005 after a decade as the division director of reproductive medicine and infertility at Brown University Alpert Medical School and Women and Infants Hospital in Providence, Rhode Island.

After graduating from Harvard College as magna cum laude in 1976, he attained a medical degree at Georgetown University in 1980. He returned to Cambridge to intern at Mount Auburn Hospital. He then relocated to Chicago where he completed a residency in psychiatry at the University of Chicago in 1985, concurrently with a fellowship in neuroendocrinology research at Northwestern University. During his psychiatry residency, he determined that he wanted to pursue a career in women's health. In 1989, he completed his second residency, in obstetrics and gynecology, at Yale University. He remained at Yale for two years as a Kennedy-Dannreuther research fellow in reproductive endocrinology from 1989 to 1991 and one year as a clinical fellow in reproductive endocrinology and infertility from 1991 to 1992 then joined the Yale faculty as an assistant professor until 1996. In 1996, he became the division director of reproductive endocrinology and infertility at Alpert Medical School in Providence, Rhode Island, before becoming the James M. Ingram professor and chairman of obstetrics and gynecology at USF in 2005.

His outstanding academic career has been framed with numerous honors and achievements. These have included recognition as the outstanding senior resident at Yale, recognition by the Science Coalition for Outstanding Research Breakthroughs for 1998, and selection in 1997 by the International Biographical Centre as one of 2,000 Outstanding People of the 20th Century. When he departed Tampa to assume the position of professor and chair of obstetrics and gynecology at New York University in 2009, he had authored or coauthored an excess of one hundred original scientific manuscripts in peer-reviewed journals and was the holder of four US patents pertinent to reproductive medicine.

Dr. Keefe had grown up as one of seven children in a large Irish-Catholic family along the shore of Massachusetts. He often recounted how his youngest sibling had been born to his mother when she was forty-seven years old. He and his wife, Candy, also had seven children. Undoubtedly, his affection for children and his own experiences as a child and parent drove his passion as a reproductive endocrinologist to help women and couples achieve a family. At a time when the subspecialty of reproductive endocrinology and infertility (REI) often placed arbitrary limits on the age which it would stop treating infertile women, Dr. Keefe was liberal in treating women of virtually any age who wanted to try.

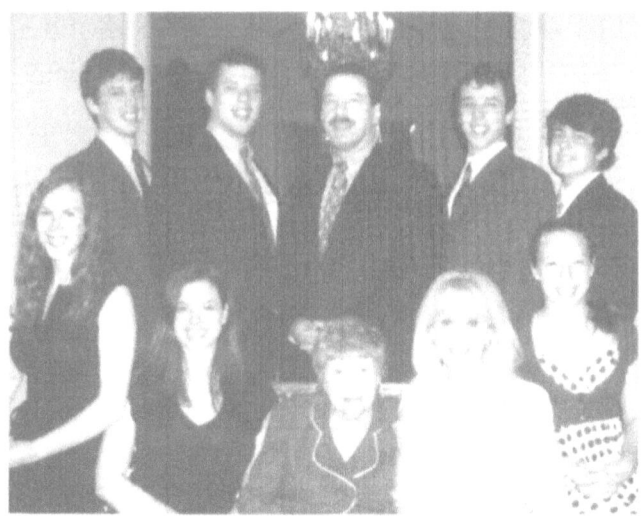

Dr. Keefe with his seven children at Thanksgiving

No doubt his mother, having his youngest sibling at age forty-seven, was Dr. Keefe's inspiration for his basic science quest to turn back the hands of time by uncovering the secrets that cause oocytes to age. With PhD colleague

Dr. Lin Lou, who came to USF with Dr. Keefe from Brown, outstanding research on oocyte segregation errors in aging oocytes during maturation and the use of telomere length as an assay of ovarian aging was undertaken. Seminal work in this arena included preliminary reports on the use of polarized-light microscopy as a noninvasive means to study the oocyte, the roles of mitochondrial DNA and oxidative stress in oocyte dysfunction, and the proposal of a "multi-hit" hypothesis reflected in shortened telomeres to explain oocyte malfunction and aging.

If Dr. Keefe's passion as a scientist was to unearth the secrets of oocyte aging, his passion as a clinician and leader was to embrace the entrepreneurial model of academic, medical health-care delivery being espoused by the USF Morsani College of Medicine under Dean Stephen Klasko, MD, MBA, during Dr. Keefe's tenure at USF from 2005 to 2009. He surrounded himself with individuals of similar entrepreneurial bent and provided them with the trust, support, guidance, and freedom to accomplish their goals.

His personality and leadership style were not authoritarian. Yet by the sheer force of the openness, trust, enthusiasm, intellect, and fundamental fairness that he exuded, he was the center of attention wherever he appeared. It was not uncommon to see Dr. Keefe and his team huddle at a table after a lecture or course, brainstorming on how to apply what had just been presented to better the USF OB-GYN Department. During those few times when he and his colleagues were together in a less formal setting (such as dinner at a conference), raucous laughter could be heard as he would recount past stories and experiences with great fanfare.

Prior to coming to Tampa, Dr. Keefe had transformed the Women and Infants Program from a mid-sized IVF program, undertaking three hundred cycles annually with average success rates, into a regional and national powerhouse with nine hundred cycles annually, fully operational IVF centers in Providence and Boston (with Tufts University School of Medicine), and excellent clinical outcomes. Following the Six Sigma Model, he had successfully broken down the IVF process unto component steps at Brown and worked with all members of the team to scrutinize and optimize each step along the way, with resulting improvement in outcome and dramatic increases in cycle volume.

At the time that he became the chairman of Obstetrics and Gynecology at USF, Dr. Keefe found kindred souls at USF Health, including the dean of USF Health, Dr. Stephen Klasko, an OB-GYN with an MBA from the University of Pennsylvania Wharton School of business. On the administrative side at USF Health and in the physicians group, Mohamad Kasti and Lou Rhodes were Six Sigma black belts who had previously worked for GE Healthcare. Dean Klasko was committed to implementing an academic entrepreneurial model of health-care delivery in the Tampa area. The medical school was in the process of expanding, not only in terms of numbers of physicians, but also programs. A state-of-the-art office building and ambulatory surgery center was being constructed in South Tampa, across from Tampa General Hospital. The confluence of academic entrepreneurialism being promoted by the dean—with an OB-GYN department that lacked some of these modern academic disciplines and needs but possessed a core nucleus of excellent faculty—proved fertile soil for expanding departmental influence as the department needed to grow; the new chairman had a proven track record for engendering growth at Brown University, and the dean was intent on seizing an opportunity to transform health care in the Tampa Bay region.

Dr. Keefe's tenure at USF was defined by the creation of a can-do attitude within the department, which resulted in overcoming many challenges. The department lacked a formal division of urogynecology, including the evolving discipline of female pelvic medicine. It lacked a comprehensive reproductive endocrinology division subsequent to Dr. Yeko having left to enter private practice in the community. It required substantial expansion of the Maternal-Fetal Medicine Division. However, the core faculty present upon his arrival was solid and committed to the growth of the department. This faculty included a strong general OB-GYN Division under the direction of Dr. Catherine Lynch, a nationally prominent USF homegrown gynecologic oncologist in Dr. Mitchel Hoffman, and a Maternal-Fetal Medicine Division shepherded by previous chairman Dr. William Spellacy and Dr. Michael Parsons, who ably served as interim chair prior to Dr. Keefe's arrival. The residency program, located at Tampa General Hospital, was on solid footing, headed as it had been for the previous years by Dr. Spellacy.

Dr. Mitchel Hoffman, who continued to head the Division of Gynecologic Oncology at Tampa General Hospital and at USF OB-GYN, collaborated with his colleagues at Moffitt for both patient care and the provision of a high-quality gynecology-oncology fellowship and continued to publish clinically relevant manuscripts in the gynecologic-oncology literature.

In order to expand the department at a time when federal Medicare funding and state Medicaid funding was tenuous and uncertain, combined with state cutbacks in financial support of the educational mission of the medical school, Dr. Keefe recognized the need to expand and diversify the Generalist Division of Obstetrics and Gynecology. He solidified Medicaid relationships and support of the resident-run Genesis Clinic but simultaneously recognized that an academic, medical department could no longer rely on the money generated by government-based programs, given the economic and political realities of the time. He worked with Dr. Lynch to essentially double the size of the Generalist Division and partitioned the division into two components.

One of these components continued to support residency training and service at the Genesis Clinic and provided resident supervision for obstetrics and gynecologic care of these patients in the hospital setting at Tampa General Hospital. The other partition developed as a private-practice model, caring for insured private patients who were exposed exclusively to board-certified or board-eligible residency graduates now on USF faculty. He further expanded the clinical umbrella of the Generalist Division by concluding a relationship with Women's Health Care, the midwife practice with contracted care for Hillsborough County Health indigent patients, whereby USF generalists became supervising physicians for the midwife group. The net result was immediate and rapid expansion in the volume of obstetrics and routine gynecology in the department.

In order to increase both the exposure and the size of the Maternal-Fetal Medicine Division, he recruited from private practice in Tampa a former residency colleague from his days at Yale, Dr. Ruben Quintero. With the collaboration and support of Tampa General Hospital, this resulted in the development of an internationally renowned fetal-surgery center. In addition, three maternal-fetal members—Dr. Quintero's spouse, Dr. Eftichia Kontopoulos; Dr. Victoria Belogolovkin; and Dr. Valerie Whiteman—were recruited, effectively more than doubling the size of the MFM Division.

To develop gynecologic urology and the new female pelvic medicine, Dr. Keefe chose as division director Dr. Lennox Hoyte. Dr. Hoyte's pedigree included a degree in engineering from MIT, a medical degree from Stanford University, and residency and fellowship training in the Harvard system. Dr. Hoyte was able to entice Dr. Stuart Hart, an Emory-trained gynecologic urologist, away from private practice in Atlanta, Georgia. Rapidly, the division surged to the forefront in developing simulation technology in gynecologic surgery, in expanding the use of robotic-assisted gynecologic surgery, in developing new medical devices for patenting, and in creating a fellowship.

It had been five years since the department had a comprehensive reproductive endocrinology division. At the time, the division was dependent for student and resident exposure in this academic discipline upon collaboration with a highly regarded prominent private practice in the community. Dr. Keefe recruited Dr. Shayne Plosker, a UCSF-trained (University of California, San Francisco) reproductive endocrinologist who had been his colleague in Providence, to become division director of the nascent Reproductive Endocrinology and Infertility Division. Drs. Keefe and

Plosker enticed Dr. Ying Ying, an embryologist with whom they had worked for many years at Brown, to leave the University of Texas at San Antonio and join them in Tampa. A year later, Dr. Celso Silva, who had undertaken his residency at Brown and subsequently a fellowship at the University of Pennsylvania, joined the team. In conjunction with Dr. James Mayer, a reproductive endocrinology and infertility program was reborn.

While there was some resistance to all this change initially, very soon, the changes energized the entire department, and growth and development took momentum on its own.

The building blocks for a successful tenure had been laid prior to Dr. Keefe's arrival through the work of Dr. Spellacy and interim chairman Dr. Michael Parsons, who had not only created a strong department and an environment conducive to positive changes, but who were extremely supportive of the new chairman upon his arrival. Both were gentlemen, offered sage advice, and contributed greatly to the success of the new chairman and continued growth of the department.

Evidence of the effect of these changes could be found in national hospital rankings reported in the *US News & World Report*, which accorded Tampa General Hospital national rankings for excellence in gynecology in 2007 and 2008.

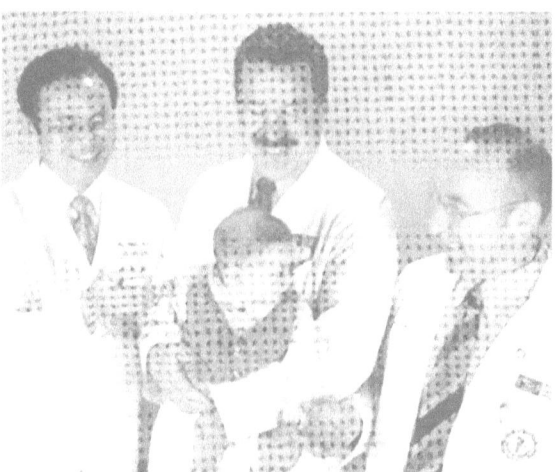

Drs. Ying, Keefe, and Plosker with a happy outcome

In four short years, the department had been transformed. After Dr. Quintero left for the University of Miami, a successful maternal-fetal-medicine nucleus has remained, and a fetal therapy center, in collaboration with Tampa General Hospital, continues to thrive. The

Urogynecology and Female Pelvic Medicine Division is providing excellent, high-volume care and continues to be an innovative leader in the field. The Generalist Division remains strong and with expanding patient volume. The IVF program, starting from ground zero, now performs over 150 cycles per year, and there are plans for an REI fellowship in the future.

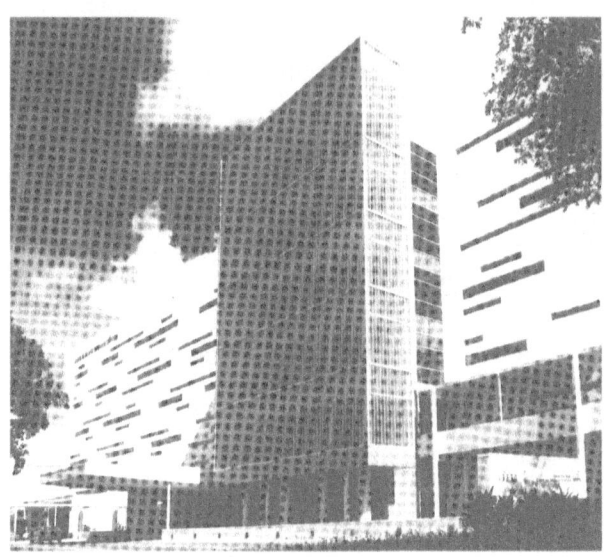

Morsani Outpatient Medical Cemter at USF, circa 2010

Dr. Keefe's tenure was not without controversy and resistance. Within the medical school and physicians group, the rapid expansion of physician numbers as well as construction of new buildings and facilities had made an investment in the future that resulted in tight finances and the need for some centralization of decision making. There were some leadership changes, but overall, the momentum created was sustainable. In 2009, Dr. Keefe departed to assume chairmanship of the Department of Obstetrics and Gynecology at New York University, but USF's Department of Obstetrics and Gynecology continued to thrive under the interim chairmanship of Dr. Catherine Lynch.

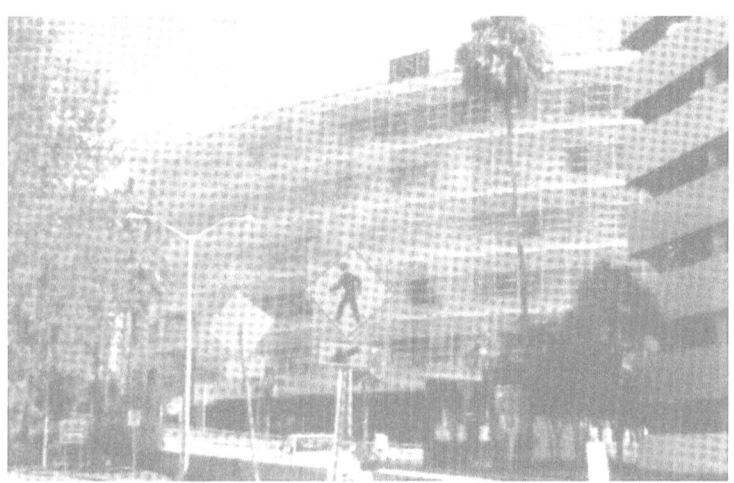

South Tampa Center for Advanced Healthcare, circa 2010

Dr. Keefe's legacy to the USF Department of Obstetrics and Gynecology was the fulfillment of his vision of creating a vibrant, creative, nurturing, secure environment. The result was a truly innovative, thriving, academic department, populated by physicians with a can-do attitude. Academic entrepreneurialism had been adopted as the way to ensure future success.

Table 12

Residents Serving under David L. Keefe, MD

Year	Resident	Medical School	
2005	Diana C. Connor, MD	U. of South Florida	
	Jennifer D. George, MD	U. of Virginia	
	Kristen E. Helm, MD	U. of Texas, Houston	
	Ryan M. Riggs, MD	U. of Oklahoma	R
	Monique N. Simmons, MD	Eastern Virginia Medical School	
2006	Nicole J. Fanarjian, MD	Albany Medical College	
	Megan D. Indermaur, MD	Saint Louis University	O
	Kirstin M. Patrick MD	Georgetown University	
	Brooke L. Slaton, MD	Emory University	
	Christine C. Tebes, MD	U. of South Florida	
2007	Evelyn G. Serrano, MD	U. of South Florida	
	Aaron B. Deutsch, MD	U. of Florida	M
	Kelly J. Hamel, MD	U. of South Florida	
	Leena J. Hancock, MD	U. of South Florida	
	Susan M. Smith, MD	U. of South Florida	F
2008	Jill C. Botelho, MD	U. of South Florida	
	Natasha K. Gooden, MD	Howard University	
	Martha E. Kapitz, MD	Indiana University	
	James M. Palmer, MD	U. of Texas Medical Branch	F
	Allison I. Ziff, MD	Medical College of Wisconsin	
2009	Elana Deutsch, MD	U. of South Florida	
	Neeraj Desai, MD	U. of California, San Diego	M
	Krista Kant, MD	U. of S. Alabama	
	Amy Sorrells, MD	U. of Texas Medical Branch	
	Natalie Yazdani, MD	Medical College of Virginia	
2010	Brian Barrow, MD	U. of Florida	
	Mona McCullough, MD	U. of Miami	U
	Quyen Nguyen, MD	U. of South Florida	

	Dawn Palaszewski, MD	SUNY Upstate, NY	F
	Pamela Twitty, MD	U. of South Florida	
2011	Siobhan Bertolino, MD	Eastern Virginia Medical School	
	Hillary Kufahl, MD	Medical College of Wisconsin	
	Karen Matta, MD	U. of South Florida	
	Jeanmarie Texier, MD	U. of South Florida	

Fellowships
O—Oncology
M—Maternal-Fetal Medicine
R—Reproductive Endocrinology and Infertility
U—Urogynecology
F—Faculty

Table 13
Faculty under David L. Keefe, MD*

Adam Urato, MD
Amanda Melina, MD
Anna Parsons, MD
Barry S. Verkauf, MD, MBA
Carol Cox, MD
Catherine Lynch, MD
Cecilia Jevitt, CNM, PhD
Celso Silva, MD
Eftichia Kontopoulos, MD
Erich Wyckoff, MD
Gerard DiLeo, MD
J. K. Williams, MD
James Burgess, MD
James Palmer, MD, MSMS
Joan McCarthy, MD
John Tsibris, PhD
Joseph Spinnato, MD
Karen Bruder, MD
Kelly Hamel, MD
Kiran Rao, MD
Larry Glazerman, MD, MBA
Lauri Hochberg, MD
Lennox Hoyte, MD, MSEE
Lin Liu, PhD
Margaret Keeling, MD
Mark McLean, PhD
Michael Parsons, MD
Mitchel Hoffman, MD
Nagwa Dajani, PhD
Nelly Levine, MD
Robyn Sayer, MD
Ruben Quintero, MD
Shayne Plosker, MD
Sheila Connery, MD
Shelly Holmstrom, MD
Stephen Kohl, MD
Stuart Hart, MD
Susan Smith, MD
Valerie Whiteman, MD
Victoria Belogolovkin, MD
William Spellacy, MD
Ying Ying, PhD
Zoi Russell, MD

---

* *In order by first name*

Introduction to Chapter 7

Adaptation to a Changing Environment

At the time this book is written, Florida obstetricians and gynecologists can take pride in a unique situation. The CEOs, vice presidents of medical or health affairs, president of health systems, and/or deans of three of Florida's medical schools are OB-GYNs: Dr. David Guzick at the University of Florida, Dr. John A. Rock at Florida International University in Miami, and Dr. Stephen K. Klasko at the University of South Florida in Tampa. All are outstanding clinicians, and each has an advanced degree in health-care administration, economics, or business administration. It appears that these latter skills are increasingly appreciated in medical executives.

Dr. Stephen Klasko was born in Pennsylvania, and his early medical career took place in Pennsylvania. A graduate of Hahnemann University Hospital and HealthEast teaching hospital residency in OB-GYN, he entered private practice in Allentown, Pennsylvania, in 1982. There he led Valley OB/GYN Associates for ten years.

In 1991, Dr. Klasko became vice chairman and residency director in the Department of Obstetrics and Gynecology at Lehigh Valley Hospital in Allentown. Having earned an MBA from the University of Pennsylvania's highly regarded Wharton School of business in 1996, he became chairman of obstetrics and gynecology at Lehigh Valley Hospital in Allentown thereafter. His teaching and clinical excellence and business acumen were readily apparent, and in 2000, he became Dean of the college of medicine at Drexel University in Philadelphia, a position he held until becoming CEO of USF Health and Dean of the Morsani College of Medicine at the University of South Florida in 2004.

While there are many subdisciplines within business, like in medicine, Dr. Klasko's niche and love is business entrepreneurship. It is the creativity demanded to find new solutions to current problems that excites him.

Health care today is in flux. While it has been said that "change is the only constant," the potential rapidity and magnitude of change that currently exists has rarely been greater. Thought leaders are hard at work on this almost certain challenge, as health-care reform is once again the buzzword about the country. In the next chapter, Dr. Klasko expresses his vision of the current and future needs required for the health of the academic community, obstetrics and gynecology as a specialty, the patients it serves, and our country at large.

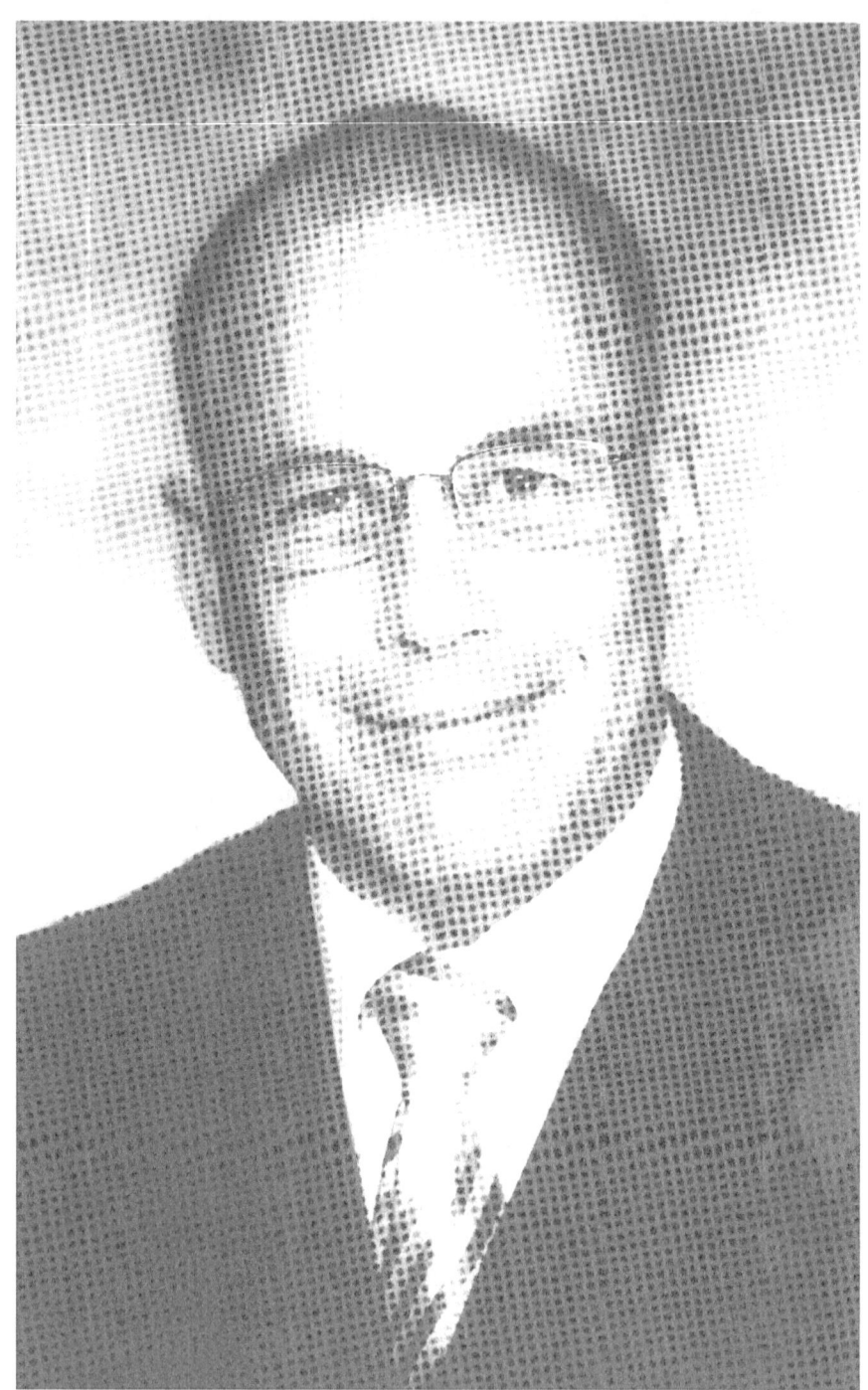

Stephen K. Klasko, MD, MBA

CHAPTER 7

What We Forgot to Teach in Medical School . . . and Why It Matters

The Unintended Consequences of the Health-Care Reform Revolution

by *Stephen K. Klasko, MD, MBA*
CEO, USF Health
Dean, Morsani College of Medicine
University of South Florida

Much energy has been expended on the exact mechanism by which health care will be reformed and whether or not it will be beneficial and, more importantly (at least to some in the debate), whom we can blame if it fails. But we have missed an essential fact. The world of academic medicine and the fragile relationship between hospital-university-practice group and even patients and students have already changed dramatically. Even in the pre-reform era, in September 2009, the economy, unemployment, and threat of major change have conspired to materially impact growth rates in most of our markets:

> Sixty-one percent of hospital facilities reported lower patient volumes, with 11 percent reporting more than a 20 percent decline.

Fifty-seven percent of academic medical centers reported a decrease in elective procedures.

For the first time in over twenty-five years, surgical procedures in the United States declined by 6 percent.

(Opinion Research Corporation Survey: Trends Impacting Healthcare Channels and the Medical Device Industry, September 2009)

Add this to the nearly historic decrease in state funding or replacement of recurrent funding with time-limited stimulus funding, and it would seem like a good time for academic medical centers to rethink some of the "sacred cows" that have haunted us in the past and make them into hamburgers. While many have chosen to wait for the white water of change to subside, the chances are that if you care enough to be proactive, sitting at the annual meeting of the AAHC, you are already one of the few that is more optimistic about the future than the past.

While we have all said it in different ways, the challenge is probably best outlined by the Institute of Medicine's Committee on Quality of Health Care in America when they stated, "the American healthcare delivery system is in need of fundamental change." The current care systems cannot do the job. Trying harder will not work. Changing systems of care will. In other words, doing the same thing that didn't work the first time and expecting different results is not a successful business strategy. Changing the DNA of health care will require a very different approach and one for which both faculty and students may need different skill sets to be prepared.

As a medical school dean and CEO of a health system that is in the midst of a transformation, I have searched for the answers to three key questions that have allowed me to be optimistic that academic medicine can thrive in Tampa and influence the community in a positive manner and that the future is indeed brighter than the past. In order to come to that conclusion, I needed to answer three questions:

Do we need to change the way we select and educate physicians?

What are the major transformations that will need to occur to avoid repeating past mistakes?

What lessons will we wish we had learned during the first decade of the millennium if we were to look back from the future?

The answers to these questions led me to five conclusions that have transformed our blueprint for strategic action at USF.

Conclusion 1: Doctors are not like other people

In an article that I cowrote for the *Physician Executive* with Richard Shel, chair of negotiations at Wharton, entitled "Biases Physicians Bring to the Table," we posited that by the way physicians have been selected and educated, we have joined a cult. That cult is based on four biases—an autonomy, competitive, hierarchal, and noncreativity bias—and that in order to change the DNA of our faculty, we will have to deprogram those biases before we can reprogram a different, more future-oriented faculty. That set of biases hinders us in collaborative negotiating, helps explain the lack of trust that often exists in a medical staff, and accounts for some of our risk aversion and unwillingness to think differently. In one part of the study, we found that 78 percent of MBAs viewed creativity as part of their success, 53 percent had a significant creative outlet such as painting or cooking, 93 percent were able to elicit examples where creativity had helped solve a major problem at work within the last year, and 85 percent routinely read books outside their field. Among physicians, only 12 percent viewed creativity as one of the major determinants of success. We had significantly fewer hobbies outside of medicine, and when we did, they often honed the same precision skills that we need in our medical career, such as flying or sailing. In essence, the number one differentiator of creativity is that MBAs *believed* they were creative, which allowed them to feel comfortable about an uncertain future and positively affected their willingness to take risk. Physicians, by and large, believed they were not. Because of that, they felt their lives were affected by external factors. Among academic physicians, a major source of pessimism was that we had become autonomous creatures losing control.

In fact, one need go no further than a comment made by a business colleague who said, "Let me get this straight. You still accept students into medical school based on science GPA, MCATs, and organic-chemistry grades, yet you're amazed that doctors are not more empathetic, communicative, and creative." In fact, in a recent survey, we asked graduating residents after a year in practice or on faculty what they wished they had learned. As it turned out, it was not more microbiology, biochemistry, or gynecology. Instead, their shortcomings included being an individual in an organization, marketing their practice, making patients happy, collaborative negotiations, and managing up. So if there was ever a time to rethink the educational mission, that time is now. At USF, we have responded in three ways:

1. *The health-care leadership track at Lehigh Valley Health Network.* The Macy Report commissioned by the AAMC in 2008 was unanimous in the view that "medical educators should seize the current call for expanded enrollment as an opportunity to make additional improvements." This report stated what we already know—namely, that we need to bring medical education into better alignment with societal needs and goals. In essence, we are still teaching physicians what they needed to know in the past, instead of preparing them for the future.

   Our goal is to take a cohort of students, select them based on leadership potential, create a four-year curriculum around the skill sets needed in the future, and then tailor their clinical clerkships and externships in such a way that the above biases will be deprogrammed from the start. During the formation of this track, it became clear to us that in order for this to be successful, we would need a hospital partner that was philosophically close to us in relation to leadership training, interprofessional education and commitment to the education, and practice of quality and safety. It also became clear that geographic proximity was probably the least important parameter. The end result was a partnership with a great hospital and community academic entity 1,150 miles away in what is now the northern academic campus of USF. This medical school track will begin admitting students in 2011—students who are selected based not only on scientific parameters, but valid emotional intelligence and leadership potential parameters, with a curriculum that will be both interprofessional and codesigned from colleagues in leadership executive education, as well as correcting the deficiencies cited above.

2. *Areas of scholarly concentration for medical students.* At USF, we have begun a program whereby every medical student must take a forty-credit hour "minor" that will expand their horizon and foster their creativity. That minor can be in business, public health, law, education, health disparities, or research. This program not only adds another area of expertise for each medical student graduating from USF, but also allows for a smoother route to dual degrees including MD/MBA, MD/JD, MD/MPH or MD/PhD.

3. *Interprofessional education.* The inability to create high-powered teams among health-care professionals is one of the obstacles to

future success in an environment where that teamwork will be a necessary component of a quality-accountable system. Over the past three years, we have made a solid commitment to training doctors, nurses, public health professionals, and pharmacists *together*. We want them to recognize how to combat the obstacles to team success, such as poor communication, lack of trust, and personality issues. Beginning in 2010, every medical student will be required to take one course in public health, pharmacy, and nursing focused around quality, safety, and epidemiology.

Conclusion 2: We need to move from SOFTIs to CRISPs

Improving the value equation in health care will require a different mind-set as it relates to departments and service lines. Unfortunately, the dialogue has been confused as definitions of service lines have often been mediated by hospital marketing executives, and the decisions surrounding their formation are often done without significant faculty involvement. As a health science center that does not own or control its own hospital, we had an opportunity to create an endowed ambulatory center of the future. We were challenged by a donor to overcome the service obstacles that are often associated with academic ambulatory care.

Planning for this center included patient, nursing, public health, and pharmacy input into the ideal patient experience. It was designed to guarantee more efficient communication. The implementation of the USF Morsani Center for Advanced Health Care allowed us to create a multidisciplinary program designed to enhance access, create more efficient care, and improve outcomes. The organizational implications of these goals required us to transform our faculty from SOFTIs (silos of full-time individuals) to CRISPs (clinical—and research-integrated strategic programs).

So each one of our providers in that building began a process of understanding what will increasingly be a truism of an entrepreneurial academic model, namely that there are two parents—the academic entity as well as the entrepreneurial multidisciplinary CRISP. In this two-paycheck model, an orthopedic surgeon will receive his/her academic payment from the Orthopedic Department, but his/her clinical incentives will be based on the success of the entire sports-medicine team, consisting of orthopedic surgeons, family physicians, physical therapists, and other sports-related providers.

This approach has had mixed success. On the one hand, this entrepreneurial approach created an unprecedented interest among the academic faculty in business development, service, and market share that resulted in patients' service guarantees; a coordinated, electronic pharmacy program; mystery shoppers to determine service lapses; and a unique cross-provider retail partnership with a regional supermarket. On the other hand, the CRISPs have been limited by inconsistency in support among clinical chairs, as well as decreased state funding, which has limited our ability to support the appropriate behavior. The next step will be to clearly demarcate the responsibility and accountability of the academic department leaders as opposed to the CRISP CEOs.

Conclusion 3: "It is difficult to get someone to understand something when their salary depends upon them not understanding it" (Upton Sinclair)

In academic medicine, on both the hospital and university side of the equation, we have been guilty of sending mixed messages as it relates to incentivizing behavior consistent with the organization's goals. Based on publicly available data, we reviewed a variety of CEO and hospital-senior-management incentives that were often inconsistent with the stated goals and vision of the health center. For example, in many cases, the board's stated goals were quality, service, national prominence, and community well-being. Yet often the CEO and his/her immediate senior managers were paid based on hospital census, net-net financials, and bond rating. It is fair to say that business principles would predict that if you want to see what the hospital will look like ten years from now, one can look at the CEO's incentive package today. There are a growing number of very innovative incentive packages that nonprofit board members are encouraging for their hospital senior executives. In these models, the medical staff/faculty is involved in senior-management incentive discussions, and those incentives are largely based on objective parameters of patient satisfaction, national prominence, balanced dashboards of objective quality data, and physician/faculty satisfaction.

At USF, we decided to embark on a bold initiative of tying faculty incentives to the organization's strategic goals. This initiative, called AIMS (asset-investment management system), involved over one hundred faculty members. It was created over three years by a council trichaired by an academic, basic science chair; an academic, clinical science chair; and an administrative chair. It has now evolved to include clinical RVUs, research productivity, and EVUs (educational value units) in what has become a faculty-directed and modified incentive system for our future. At the same time, we initiated a web-based system and approved the purchase of a health-data repository entitled HART (health analytical reporting and tracking), which extracts and stores performance data from the many data sources within the academic medical center and university. This real-time, all-source mechanism allows a faculty member to understand exactly what his/her goals are, separate those goals into their academic and business components, and be able to assess in real time their potential for incentive payment or salary adjustment. This flexibility, real-time reporting, and continuous communication with the faculty has been a major driver in promoting the culture change necessary to maintain the entrepreneurial academic model.

Academic medicine is an extraordinarily complex environment, and incentive systems have often had unintended, sometimes mission-counter consequences. The most recent addition to AIMS will be a comprehensive, data-driven, and mission-based EVU model that will ensure faculty are given appropriate credit for their instructional effort in undergraduate medical education, graduate medical education, and graduate education (master's and PhD). Faculty who are assigned to major teaching or leadership roles or essential, educational, administration activities that exceed our 5 percent minimum standards will be provided with EVU credit that translates into salary and released time to enable them to fulfill their assigned duties. Data will also be collected on faculty achievement of excellence in performance benchmarks related to these assigned roles. Faculty members' achievement of benchmarks will guide discretionary bonuses and support tenure and promotions decisions.

Conclusion 4: Process drives culture, and building a performance culture requires leadership development, mentoring, and succession planning

There has been increasing interest in leadership training for faculty senior managers as well as academic leaders, but are we even targeting the people who will lead the cultural transformation? Through my work at the Governance Institute, surveying over fifty CMOs and VPMAs, there is an almost uncannily consistent distribution of faculty/medical staff and their attitude toward the organization's leadership. In round terms, there was a mean of 20 percent of the medical staff who consistently and vocally supported the leadership, 15 percent who represented a vocal minority of naysayers, and a relatively silent majority among the rest of the faculty. In these organizations, we found that the CMO/dean spent much of their time on the "converted," way too much time frustrating themselves trying to "heal" the disenfranchised, and the least amount of time on the segment that can make the largest impact on cultural transformation—the nearly silent majority.

We believe that the transformation of the organization starts with changing the leadership culture one leader or potential leader at a time. In essence, we needed to change the DNA of our medical school. So, in 2005, USF created a Center for Transformation and Innovation (CTI). Its charge was to accelerate the vision of USF Health by transforming the leadership DNA at all levels within the organization, including students. The goal was to develop leaders through a systematic succession planning and talent-management process, providing the necessary skills through leadership development, removing disincentives, and shifting beliefs. This center created a path to physician leadership development through a model program, the Leadership Institute at USF Health, designed to promote a culture of leadership excellence and success.

The Leadership Institute at USF Health guides participants through cultural and leadership challenges in a way that builds our organization's core vision—transforming how health care is delivered and how health is understood in a continuum from the environment, to the community, then to the individual. To achieve this transformation, we enhanced the tools of leadership—leading with strategy, leading people, and leading for results—with the four-year goal of converting over one hundred medical staff/faculty members to leadership and strategically aligned roles in the organization. This center created a path to physician leadership, which included creating the right environment, developing leaders in a way that met our goals.

The succession-planning program at USF Health is a deliberate and systematic effort to ensure leadership continuity in key positions and to encourage individual advancement. The Leadership Institute at USF Health focuses on those professionals who demonstrate high leadership potential within USF Health and are already making a positive difference within the organization. The foundation premise of top-level leadership development is that leaders are not simply born, but are created through life experiences, reflection, and learning.

The health-care industry may be unique in the enormity of the talent challenges that confront it. If there were ever a perfect storm related to succession development and talent management, it is most acute in health care, according to Allan Schweyer, Human Capital Institute ("The State of Talent Management in the Healthcare Industry" by Allan Schweyer, Human Capital Institute in partnership with Lawson Software, May 2009). He goes on to say that while it is true that the aging population restricts talent for all industries, it is only in health care and life sciences that it so profoundly impacts demand at the same time. To prepare, he suggests that health-care organizations

1. build and maintain a strong employer brand and cooperate to build a strong brand for the industry,
2. develop strategic and ongoing succession planning and development processes,
3. create strategic recruitment plans and develop a variety of creative tools to attract top talent,
4. build effective on-boarding and mentoring programs and processes,
5. create great places to work so that the top talent will remain with health-care organizations,
6. identify and develop leaders at all levels and dedicate the resources necessary to accomplish and sustain leadership development throughout the organization and over time,
7. communicate and manage your plan effectively, and
8. reward talent with strategic employee recognition.

Our Center for Transformation and Innovation has allowed us to merge the appropriate, bold, corporate best practices into our academic environment to confront these talent challenges that have been and will continue to be a major driver of culture change in our organization.

Conclusion 5: "We tend to overestimate technology in the short term and underestimate it in the long term" (Roy Amara)

At USF, as at many other academic medical centers, we have patted ourselves on the back for converting to electronic medical records and utilizing today's technology effectively. But in many cases, we have not understood the extent of the long-term changes that will occur with the combustion of a new wave of consumer technologies, as well as the gap between the electronic and technologic footprint of the senior managers as compared to the generation represented by our students and younger patients.

The pace is revealing. The number of health-related web sites in the past two years has increased by one hundredfold. The number of people under age forty that said they get a significant amount of health information online has increased by tenfold. Google, Microsoft, and Yahoo have stated that they view health care as their number-one revenue opportunity, and one of the fastest-growing segments of health care—medical tourism—is marketed almost exclusively online.

In a recent survey that I conducted, it became increasingly evident that patients and students under age thirty-five expect health care to be a consumer sport in the near future.

> Seventy-one percent expect that their doctor's visits would have online scheduling with comparative rates by 2011.

> Eighty-three percent expect that within two years, they will be able to access their health records with the same ease in which they view their online accounts.

> Eighty-five percent expect that there will be social networking opportunities to discuss health-related topics and compare providers.

> Ninety-two percent expect to have two-way electronic communication with their providers.

At USF Health, we have embarked on an extreme technologic makeover that includes the following:

1. *PaperFree Tampa Bay*—A federally funded program in which we partner with the colleges of education, engineering, and communication to recruit and train electronic health-care ambassadors, a group of vendor-agnostic missionaries whose goal is to transform an entire ten-county region to an electronic health-record environment. The federal funding is being used to create a curriculum, hire and train health-care ambassadors, create consumer awareness, and accomplish the goals of 100 percent of physicians using e-prescribing as well as providing them decision support for electronic health records. The University of South Florida will demonstrate to the nation that we will build a clear and measurable IT infrastructure for a community-based electronic prescribing system within health practitioners' offices throughout this ten-county area.

2. *Assessment of technical competence through a center for advanced medical learning and simulation.* The center will be a world-class, state-of-the-art medical-conference facility that

will house an approximately fifty-six thousand square-foot real-life working-and-teaching environment. It will be located in a secured, controlled-access area equipped with advanced technology to facilitate the transfer of knowledge and skills to the learner. In addition to being a sophisticated training center, it will also include two research and development components. One is the concept laboratory for prototype development and testing of new techniques and technologies in robotic, computer-assisted, and image-guided surgery. Another is the educational research component, which will house researchers and staff who will examine and test educational practices to assist faculty, staff, and students in applying knowledge and technology to produce valid and innovative education for health-care professionals. We will be partnering with leaders in flight simulation, as well as industry leaders, to create valid means and standard deviations of technical competence on the road to valid simulation-based credentialing and quality training.

3. *Partnership with Apple Inc. through a leadership symposium in digital health care.* A steering committee was created with thought leaders in the use of digital media in health care and health-care education, including health-science representatives from USF, MD Anderson Cancer Center, Duke University, Medical College of Georgia, and the University of Michigan. This created a national conversation on how to leverage technology and mobile devices to increase access to health-care curricula. These discussions of e-learning environments, learning knowledge centers, and effective use of digital media education have created a unique opportunity to have a public-private dialogue of changes in technology as well as teaching strategies and skill sets that will be necessary for a very different future.

4. *Emerging technologies such as human RFID, Second Life, and closed-loop EMR malpractice-mitigation modules.*

In 2006, a member of the president's cabinet said this about our military future: "There are known knowns. These are things we know that we know. There are known unknowns. That is to say, these are things we know we don't know. But there are also unknown unknowns. These are things we don't know we don't know." Whether or not that was accurate from a military point of view, it could be a signpost for the future of university-hospital relationships in the current, uncertain health-care future.

We *know* that the economic and political pressures currently driving the health-care-reform debate will stress the already fragile economic and strategic partnerships in academic medicine between hospitals, universities, and physician faculty. We *know* that we *don't know* how the cost, access, quality changes, and mandates will affect our traditional clinical, research, educational, and academic missions. Will it create a den of piranhas—a new era of animosity and distributive negotiating between the traditional components of academic medical centers? Or will it create a tropical aquarium whereby these extreme pressures force an era of collaboration and overcome the competitive, hierarchal, autonomous, and noncreative biases to which we have traditionally fallen victim? At USF Health, we *don't know* the answer to that, but we *do know* that:

- *the training of new health-care leaders;*
- *the movement toward integrated, strategic partnerships between faculty of different departments and colleges;*
- *incentive programs that are faculty driven and reflect the new definitions of academic excellence and collaboration;*
- *changing the DNA of academic health care through fostering creativity in an entrepreneurial-academic model, leadership training, and succession planning;*
- *and the development and employment of new technologies to better serve our students and patients*
- will help us create an environment whereby each component of our academic medical center is bringing us closer to an optimistic future for ourselves and the Greater Tampa Bay community.

At USF, as an organization, we have taken a leadership role in moving academic health centers in advance of and beyond what any legislation can provide. At USF Health, we believe that focusing on our greatest asset, our people, will be the differentiating factor in making that change. We found that creating the incentives and exciting the people in the organization who "get it" were the motivating factors to change.

While Congress is discussing the concept of the creation of health-innovation zones, our nation's academic health centers have the opportunity to lead that charge. Our ability to boldly lead in an entrepreneurial, academic, and interdisciplinary manner will require a change in our traditional academic medical culture. Culture change is often a long and painful process. At USF Health, we have shortened that process by creating a sense of urgency, pulling together the guiding team, developing the culture-change vision and strategy, communicating for understanding and buy-in, empowering others to act, producing short-term wins, and not letting up.

Epilogue

Two things prompt my adding this epilogue. While this book has principally focused on the departmental chairmen who have led this department over the past forty years, many others have made significant contributions to both its stability and growth. Between chairmen, there always seems to be a hiatus. A search committee is appointed to look for the next chairman while an interim "chairman" is appointed to "ballast the ship" until a new chairman is found. Three important people served this role over that forty-year interval. From the time Dr. Ingram stepped down as chairman until Dr. Spellacy arrived, Dr. Denis Cavanagh served as interim chairman, and between the interval of Dr. Spellacy stepping down as chairman and the arrival of Dr. Keefe, Dr. Michael Parsons skillfully guided the department. Dr. Keefe's departure resulted in the interim chairmanship of Dr. Catherine Lynch, who ably provided her leadership skills during an interval exceeding a year. These three people are deserving of special mention for their efforts.

In addition, recently a new—and only the fourth—chairman of the department has been named. He is Dr. Jerome Yankowitz, a maternal-fetal medicine specialist, who led that division at the University of Iowa over the last seventeen years. Uniquely, Dr. Yankowitz is also a diplomate of the American Board of Medical Genetics. Dr. Yankowitz was chosen after an intense and competitive search, and we look forward to long, productive years of leadership as medicine enters perhaps its most tumultuous times in recent history.

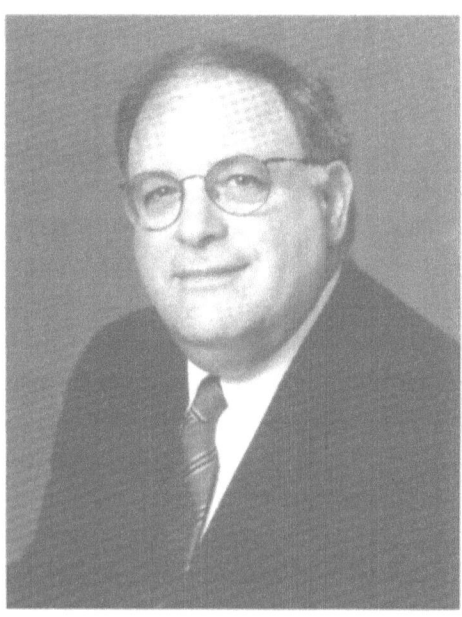

Barry S. Verkauf received his MD degree from Tulane University and completed his obstetrics-and-gynecology residency and fellowship training in reproductive endocrinology and infertility at the Johns Hopkins Hospital. In 1997, he completed the MBA program for physicians at the University of South Florida College of Business Administration. A member of the charter faculty of the Morsani College of Medicine at USF, he subsequently entered private practice in Tampa for thirty years. He currently is a professor in the Division of Reproductive Endocrinology and Infertility at the University of South Florida.

The health-care industry and its professional practice are currently in uncertain times as the outcome of the hotly debated health-care reform is awaited. While the magnitude of potential change may be unchallenged, the past century has been one of continual change for the medical profession and its practice. The rapidity of this change has continually increased with emerging new technologies and changes in the social fabric of society. Even the doctor-patient relationship has changed.

Medicine as a profession and the specialties within it have had to adapt to this change in order to be relevant to the physicians it trains, the patients they treat, and to maintain status among their peers. This book chronicles the history of the successful adaptation to required changes in one medical-school department.

INDEX